Maternal Physiology

Maternal Physiology

Tom Lind, MB, BS, PhD
Medical Research Council
Human Reproduction Group
Princess Mary Maternity Hospital
Newcastle Upon Tyne
England

CREOG

Basic Science Monograph in Obstetrics and Gynecology

Council on Resident Education in Obstetrics and Gynecology
600 Maryland Avenue, SW, Washington DC 20024-2588

Library of Congress Cataloging in Publication Data

Lind, Tom, 1934-
  Maternal physiology.

  (Basic science monograph in obstetrics and gyne-
cology)
  Bibliography: p.
  Includes index.
  1. Pregnancy. 2. Women—Physiology.
I. Title.   II. Series.
RG556.L55   1985   612'.6   84-23058
ISBN 0-915473-03-8

**The development of this Basic Science Monograph
in Maternal Physiology was made possible by a
grant from Parke-Davis.**

Contents

Preface

Modern medical practice is characterized by the degree to which it is based on scientific fact. Practice by intuition or anecdotal experiences, which may have been laudable at one point in medical history, is now condemned because it cannot withstand, or is not subjected to, the scrutiny of "scientific method." Therefore, the quality of a physician's practice is greatly influenced by the extent of the individual's scientific knowledge.

Medical education reflects a marked heterogeneity—in both the academic setting of medical school and the clinical orientation of residency programs. Today's rapid pace of scientific discoveries has an impact on the practice of obstetrics and gynecology. This fact dictates the continuing identification of basic science information most pertinent to the specialty.

In response to this need, the Council on Residency Education in Obstetrics and Gynecology (CREOG), under the direction of the CREOG Committee on Education and Curriculum, has developed a series of basic science monographs. These monographs are designed to review principles related to, but not necessarily clinically correlated with, direct patient care. The information in this series has been carefully selected to form a foundation for the application of basic science principles in a clinical environment. Such a background is an essential part of postgraduate education—both in residency and in continuing medical education.

Intentionally, the monographs are neither all encompassing nor exhaustively detailed; textbooks and other reference sources are available for more in-depth study. Rather, the review of basic science as reflected in this monograph series serves as a basis for discussion, amplification, and exploration of information particularly relevant to reproductive health. The content will be reviewed periodically and, based on critiques and feedback received, revised to ensure currency and applicability to the specialty.

To enhance the authoritativeness and usefulness of the monographs, specialists well versed in their respective fields were invited to serve as authors. CREOG is indebted to Tom Lind, PhD, for writing the text of this monograph on *Maternal Physiology,* which in six chapters, outlined and indexed in detail with succinct summarizations preceding each chapter, provides an overview of the physiologic dynamics of pregnancy.

Foreword

More than a million years of evolution have determined the optimal physiologic conditions necessary for our bodies to work efficiently. This internal environment, or "milieu interieur" as Claude Bernard more elegantly described it, is rigorously controlled. For example, the hydrogen ion concentration of our blood is maintained at pH 7.4, our plasma sodium concentration around 135 mEq/liter, and our plasma osmolality about 290 mosm/kg. Highly complex systems have evolved to maintain this homeostasis, and any sustained deviation from the normal range of values usually indicates the presence of some pathologic condition. There is one major exception, however—normal pregnancy.

The physiologic status of a normal, healthy pregnant woman changes as her pregnancy advances. Many of these changes are of such magnitude that the unwary obstetrician may diagnose disease in a patient who is only displaying the extremes of physiologic adaptation. For example, serum urea decreases by about 30%, creatinine clearance increases by about 50%, and serum progesterone can increase 1,000-fold. These progressive changes in biochemical and endocrinologic values cannot be optimum for the physiologic functioning of the mother and, teleologically at least, must be to the advantage of her developing fetus.

The first aim of this book is to describe the major maternal adaptations that occur throughout pregnancy; without a complete understanding of these normal changes, we cannot hope to clarify the causes of the many complications that can affect the expectant mother and her developing child.

Modern clinicians, whatever their specialty, rely to an increasing extent on the results obtained from laboratory tests for the management of their patients; for some, deviation from an accepted range of laboratory values is in itself sufficient to warrant treatment. Clinical management on this basis alone implies a confidence in the "normality" of any reported range of values that is seldom justified, however, particularly in regard to the expectant mother. Ideally, pregnancy-specific normal values would be determined from studies of healthy women with certain menstrual dates who have trouble-free pregnancies that result in live, healthy, and well-grown babies at term. A large number of observations should be made at each stage of gestation, under standardized conditions, and with reliable laboratory methods. Unfortunately, such data are rare, and the ranges considered normal for males and nonpregnant females are usually applied to the clinical management of pregnant women.

The second aim of this book is to make the reader aware of the need to use pregnancy-specific laboratory ranges whenever possible. When such data are not available, the obstetrician should determine them and publish them for the benefit of all—bearing in mind the strict criteria that must be applied for the collection of such information.

Many of the data discussed in this book derive from the work of my own team, because we adhered to the criteria outlined as far as possible and the biochemical and endocrinologic determinations were undertaken in our own laboratories. Many gaps remain in our understanding of pregnancy, however, and it is hoped that some readers will be stimulated to undertake the necessary research to provide the answers.

The format has been designed with the needs of those studying for examinations in mind. Each chapter begins with a summary of the major physiologic changes that affect the system under discussion; the details are then expanded in the text. At first reading, the summary will not be particularly informative, and the first-time reader should concentrate on the text. Once the facts have been absorbed, however, and under the pressure of upcoming examinations, it is hoped that the summary will become a useful aide-memoire.

T. L.

1
Volume and Composition of Blood

HEMATOLOGIC SYSTEM

Plasma volume
> *Increases* by 40% to 60% between 12 and 36 weeks of gestation.

Total erythrocyte volume
> *Increases* progressively to values some 15% above nonpregnancy values in women not taking iron supplementation, but 30% above those values in iron-supplemented patients.

Hematocrit
> By 36 weeks' gestation has *decreased* by approximately 5% in those not given iron, but only 3% in those given iron.

Hemoglobin concentration
> By last trimester, has *decreased* some 10% below nonpregnancy levels in those not taking iron, but only 2% below those levels, on average, in those taking iron.

Erythrocyte count
> *Decreases* to reach a nadir between 26 and 30 weeks some 12% below nonpregnancy values whether iron is taken or not. Values tend to increase slightly thereafter, being only 8% lower by term.

Mean cell volume
> Volume of individual red cells *increases* slightly in women not taking iron, but increase is significantly greater in those taking iron supplements.

Erythrocyte sedimentation rate
> *Considerably increased* such that it is of little diagnostic value during pregnancy.

Erythrocyte fragility
Red cells *more fragile* during pregnancy (i.e., less able to stand an decrease in osmolality).

White cell count
Increases by about 8% toward term and appears to be unaffected by iron supplementation. This is due largely to an increase in the number of neutrophils; there is little change in the eosinophil and lymphocyte counts, but the platelet count is decreased slightly.

Serum iron
Decreases by approximately 35% toward term, but shows considerable variation among individuals. This decrease is also evident in those taking iron, but to a smaller extent.

Serum transferrin
Increases by 100% or more by the second trimester. Total iron-binding capacity *increases* by 25% to 100%.

Serum ferritin
Decreases markedly, reaching a nadir during the second trimester whether or not iron supplements are taken. Values 30% or less of the nonpregnancy average are common.

Red cell protoporphyrin
Increases during normal pregnancy from approximately 0.25 mg/liter to 0.35 mg/liter erythrocytes.

Blood glucose
Fasting level *decreases* in first trimester and does not change thereafter; postprandial levels remain elevated longer during pregnancy, thereby prolonging the return to the fasting value.

Plasma folate
Decreases by approximately 50% toward term, but there is a wide range of values among individuals.

Red cell folate
Decreases slightly during pregnancy, but much less marked than the plasma decrease.

Vitamin B_{12}
Decreases in red cells and serum by 50% or more. Plasma binding capacity increases due to raised levels of transcobalamin II.

Erythropoietin
Increases about fourfold, but wide individual variations.

Anemia
Difficult to diagnose; laboratory findings must be judged by pregnancy-specific standards.

Blood viscosity

Decreases from a value of 4.61 to 3.84 relative to distilled water by 28 weeks' gestation.

BIOCHEMICAL AND GENERAL COMPOSITION OF SERUM AND PLASMA

Osmolality

Decreases by about 10 mosm/kg during first trimester and stable thereafter. Decrease in colloid osmotic pressure is similar.

Electrolytes

Sodium: Decreases during early pregnancy by about 3 mEq/liter and stable thereafter.

Potassium: Decreases by about 0.5 mEq/liter in a pattern similar to that of sodium.

Calcium: Both total and ionized calcium *decrease* by a small amount.

Magnesium: Decreases between 10% and 20% during the first half of pregnancy, with a possible small increase toward term.

Zinc: Decreases in a pattern similar to that of magnesium.

Copper: Increases from about 1.14 mg/liter to 2.03 mg/liter by term.

Chloride: Little change, if any.

Bicarbonate: Decreases markedly, probably to compensate for the decrease in P_{CO_2}.

Phosphate: Little change, if any.

Proteins

Total protein: Decreases from about 72 g/liter to 62 g/liter, with the major change occurring during the first trimester.

Albumin: Decreases from about 47 g/liter to 36 g/liter in a pattern similar to that of total protein concentrations.

Globulin: Increases from about 25 g/liter to 27 g/liter, but is a complex of increases and decreases in the various globulin fractions.

Maternal α-fetoprotein: Increases during pregnancy, particularly in women with an intrauterine death.

Enzymes

Lactate dehydrogenase, isocitrate dehydrogenase (ICDH) and α-hydroxybutyrate dehydrogenase: Unchanged from the nonpregnancy ranges.

17β-Hydroxysteroid oxidoreductase: Increases progressively from about 20 weeks' gestation to term.

Monoamine oxidase: Appears to be *unchanged* by pregnancy.

Diamine oxidase: Increases about twofold by term.

Ceruloplasmin: Increases to about double the nonpregnancy mean by term.

Glutamatic-oxalacetic transaminase (GOT) and glutamatic-pyruvic transaminase (GPT): Unchanged by pregnancy.

Creatine kinase: Decreases during the first half of pregnancy.

Lipase: Markedly reduced during normal pregnancy.

Pseudocholinesterase: Appears to be *decreased* during normal pregnancy.

Alkaline phosphatase: Increases during pregnancy because of the presence of a heat-stable fraction formed in the placenta.

Acid phosphatase: Essentially *unchanged.*

α-Amylase (diastase): Appears to be *unchanged.*

Cystine aminopeptidase and leucine aminopeptidase: Both *increase* progressively during the second and third trimesters.

Lipids

Total lipids: Taking these heterogeneous compounds as a whole, *increase* progressively.

Triglycerides: Increase progressively.

Cholesterol: Increases progressively to term.

Phospholipids: Increase progressively to term.

Nonesterified ("free") fatty acids: Overall *increase* throughout pregnancy.

Nonprotein Nitrogen

Urea: Decreases markedly during the first trimester, *stabilizes* during the second, and *increases* slightly toward term.

Creatinine: Decreases, then *increases* in a pattern similar to that of urea.

Amino acids: Various changes, some increasing while others remain unchanged or decrease.

Uric acid: Decreases markedly during the first trimester, the pattern of change being similar to those of urea and creatinine.

Vitamins

Ascorbic acid: Varies considerably, depending on dietary intake, but fasting levels may decrease somewhat.

B_6: *Decreases* quite markedly throughout pregnancy.

Clotting Factors

Fibrinogen (Factor I): Increases by about 2 g/liter by term.

Factors VII, VIII, and X: Increase during pregnancy.

Factors IX and XII: Increase somewhat in activity.

Factors XI and XIII: Decrease by 30% or more by term.

Antithrombin III (anti-Xa): Thought to be *decreased.*

Fibrin and fibrinogen degradation products: Increase progressively throughout pregnancy.

The measurements most commonly requested in the clinical management of patients are those concerned with blood. Examining a sample of blood, usually obtained from an antecubital vein, provides only a pale reflection of internal events, however. Therefore, it is necessary to understand the physiologic adaptations that affect the composition of blood during the course of normal pregnancy in healthy women in order to understand and interpret correctly the "routine" laboratory investigations so regularly requested.

Hematologic System

PLASMA VOLUME

The volume of the total vascular bed increases during pregnancy. The extra blood flow to the uterus is a major contributor to this space, as is the increased blood flow to the skin that allows the pregnant woman to radiate away the additional heat generated by her higher basal metabolic rate. Organ perfusion generally improves, particularly to the kidneys, although animal data suggest that blood flow to the liver and to skeletal muscle is not increased. When accurately weighed amounts of Evans blue dye were used to study plasma volume in a group of 36 healthy women before they became pregnant and at regular intervals throughout their subsequent pregnancies (Table 1–1), no relation was found between the incremental increase in plasma volume and the individuals' prepregnancy starting values, height, or weight. While most women reached their highest recorded value at 36 weeks of gestation, some attained it as early as 28 weeks and maintained that level until at least 36 weeks.

There is some controversy in the literature regarding a possible decrease in plasma volume between 36 weeks of gestation and term. Some authors suggest that the decrease is "real," while others believe it to be an artifact caused by posture. Certainly, in most studies that show a decrease in volume during this time, the

Table 1-1. *Plasma volume (ml) throughout pregnancy in 36 healthy women (primiparous and multiparous) having uncomplicated pregnancies and normal infants at term*

	Gestation (weeks)					
Prepregnancy	*6*	*12*	*20*	*28*	*36*	*38*
2297	2423	2470	3160	3586	3652	3615
± 278*	± 250	± 306	± 330	± 440	± 501	± 542

* ± 1 SD

tests were performed while the patients were lying supine and pressure of the uterus on the inferior vena cava could have impeded mixing of the dye. In our series of patients studied from 28 weeks of gestation onward, the patients were asked to lie on their left side as soon as the dye had been injected; despite this, some of the women displayed a small reduction in plasma volume between 36 and 38 weeks, while others did not. It seems reasonable to conclude that responses vary widely among individuals. Although a few individuals display a small and clinically insignificant decrease in this period, the highest values are usually achieved about 36 weeks of pregnancy and maintained to term. It is unusual for patients to show a progressive increase in volume until term.

Some reports suggest that the magnitude of the plasma volume increase is related to reproductive efficiency, usually defined in terms of the infant's birthweight. Such a contention is difficult to prove unless all the other variables known to affect birthweight, such as maternal stature, parity, and fetal sex, are taken into account. In this and other series, the correlation coefficient between maximum plasma volume and infant birthweight was $r = 0.44$ ($n = 36$), which is statistically significant but indicates only that approximately 16% of an infant's birthweight can be explained by maternal plasma volume increase. When the patients were grouped by parity, the mean increase in plasma volume was found to be greater in multiparous than primiparous women. The variation among individuals was so large, however, that such generalizations can have little clinical significance.

Multiple pregnancies have been shown to be associated with increased plasma volume. Most available data are concerned with twin pregnancies, in which peak values 70% or more above values in nonpregnant women have been recorded. There are fewer data from triplet and quadruplet pregnancies, but those available suggest that volume increases of 100% can occur. In two triplet pregnancies studied in our series, total volumes in excess of 5,000 ml (representing 120% increase) were recorded at 36 weeks of gestation.

TOTAL ERYTHROCYTE VOLUME

Two major techniques are commonly used to determine total erythrocyte volume, or red cell mass. Maternal red cells may be labeled with radioactive isotopes in vitro and injected back into the mother; the most popular tracers have been chromium 51 or phosphorus 32. There are reservations about the use of radioactive isotopes for serial determinations of total erythrocyte volume, however, and such information has usually been estimated on the basis of plasma volume and hematocrit. This indirect technique has two disadvantages: first, it is difficult to measure hematocrit accurately by centrifugation; second, the hematocrit of blood taken from an arm vein is higher than that of the blood in major or core vessels. The first difficulty has been overcome by the development of automatic blood cell counters in which hematocrit is accurately determined from the red cell count and mean cell volume. The second difficulty is usually overcome by assuming the whole body hematocrit to be 0.88 of the normal venous hematocrit. Even if the exact value to be used for whole body hematocrit is open to discussion, the application of a standard factor to all patients throughout pregnancy makes it possible to describe the relative changes in total erythrocyte volume.

By means of the latter technique, the total erythrocyte volume was determined in the same 36 women who participated in the study described earlier, at the same stages of pregnancy (Table 1–2). These patients were not given iron supplementation at any time. Thus, in general terms, the total erythrocyte volume increases by up to 25%, while plasma volume can increase by 50% or more.

In a different study conducted to determine the effect of iron supplementation on pregnant women, 45 healthy volunteers were randomly allocated into two groups. One group received a daily supplement of 325 mg ferrous sulfate plus 350 μg folic acid, while the other group received no supplement of any kind. Plasma volume and hematocrit were measured during the 12th and 36th week of pregnancy; the values 6 months postpartum were used as the nonpregnancy values. Interestingly, these data showed that a small but statistically significant decrease in the total erythrocyte volume occurred at 12 weeks (Table 1–3) and that this was not a dilutional effect of the increase in plasma volume. Cardiac output has increased by the end of the first trimester, which increases oxygen delivery to the tissues. It could be argued that this increased oxygenation mildly suppresses erythropoiesis during the first trimester of pregnancy, but that red cell production is later stimulated and the total erythrocyte volume increases; such an argument must be speculative, however, until more data are available. The important facts are that the total erythrocyte volume increases steadily with or without iron supplementation and that this increase is independent of changes in plasma volume. If pregnant women take regular iron supplementation, their total erythrocyte volume will be even greater by term.

Table 1-2. *Total erythrocyte volume (ml) for 36 patients described in Table 1-1*

	Gestation (weeks)					
Prepregnancy	6	12	20	28	36	38
1199 ± 134	1212 ± 142	1242 ± 152	1344 ± 140	1404 ± 184	1461 ± 180	1509 ± 285

Table 1-3. *Total erythrocyte volume (ml) with and without iron and folic acid supplementation between 12 weeks of gestation and term*

	Nonpregnant	Gestation (weeks)	
		12	*36*
No therapy group	1240	1138	1420
(*n* = 24)	± 146	± 136	± 181
Therapy group	1256	1159	1605
(*n* = 21)	± 141	± 136	± 221

HEMATOCRIT

Prior to the introduction of modern electronic blood cell counters, hematocrit was determined by centrifuging blood in capillary tubes and expressing the length of the column of packed blood cells as a percentage of the total length of the fluid column. Results obtained on different occasions often varied, however, because of differences in the centrifugation speeds used, in the time the sample was exposed to this g force, and in the internal diameter along the length of any given glass capillary tube. Such variations are no longer problems because hematocrit is now calculated from the red cell count and mean cell volume.

The 36 women described earlier showed a progressive decrease in hematocrit throughout pregnancy (Table 1–4), which reflects the balance between the increase in plasma volume and the maintenance of or slight increase in the volume of red cells. In a separate study, 100 women were randomly allocated to two groups; one group was given the iron and folic acid supplement described earlier, and the other was given no supplement at all. By term, the mean hematocrit was 33.85% (0.3385 liter/liter) in the nonsupplemented group, but 37.09% (0.3709 liter/liter) in the supplemented group, reflecting an increase in both red cell count and mean cell volume in the latter group.

HEMOGLOBIN CONCENTRATION

No aspect of maternal physiologic adaptation to pregnancy has been more misunderstood than the decrease that occurs in hemoglobin concentration. In the 36 women studied serially (who did not receive iron), hemoglobin concentration decreased from a mean prepregnancy value of 13.4 g/dl to a 38-week concentration of 11 g/dl (Table 1–5). In a separate study of 200 women, hemoglobin values decreased in *both* those women who received iron and those who did not until approximately 26 to 30 weeks of gestation. The concentrations increased thereafter

Table 1-4. *Hematocrit throughout pregnancy in the 36 women described in Table 1–1*

Gestation (weeks)	Hematocrit (%)
Prepregnancy	38.73
4	37.96
6	37.65
8	36.98
10	36.75
12	35.95
16	35.13
20	33.91
24	32.55
28	32.28
32	32.33
36	32.32
38	33.12

in those given supplements, however; by term, their values had almost returned to the prepregnancy average (Table 1–6). Hence, the hemoglobin concentration decreases during pregnancy to a new and lower value that is usually maintained until term, but iron supplementation restores the concentration to an almost "normal" level.

ERYTHROCYTE COUNT

Like the hemoglobin concentration, the erythrocyte count decreases during pregnancy. From a prepregnancy average of $4.35 \times 10^6/\mu l$, the erythrocyte count falls to $3.85 \times 10^6/\mu l$ in those not given iron and 4.03 in those given supplements. Again, the count appears to decrease in both groups until about 26 to 30 weeks of gestation, but the taking of oral iron causes a small increase in the count toward

Table 1-5. *Mean hemoglobin concentrations (g/dl) throughout pregnancy in 36 women not given iron or folic acid supplements*

Non-pregnant	Gestation (weeks)											
	4	6	8	10	12	16	20	24	28	32	36	38
13.4	13	12.9	12.8	12.7	12.5	12.2	11.7	11.3	11.0	10.9	10.8	11.0

Table 1-6. *Mean hemoglobin concentrations (g/dl) throughout pregnancy with and without iron supplementation*

Treatment	Gestation (weeks)						
	6–15	26–30	31–32	33–34	35–36	37–38	39+
Iron (*n* = 97)	12.4	11.4	11.6	11.8	11.7	12.0	12.2
No iron (*n* = 105)	12.2	11.2	11.1	11.0	11.0	11.0	11.1

term. This has interesting implications for iron therapy: if hemoglobin concentrations are increased while the total red cell count remains the same, more hemoglobin must be carried per red cell and cell size must therefore increase.

MEAN CELL VOLUME

From a prepregnancy average of 84.6 μm^3 (84.6 fl), the mean cell volume of individual red cells remains virtually unchanged throughout pregnancy in women not given iron. If regular iron supplements are taken, however, the mean cell volume increases progressively to an average value of 89.7 μm^3 (89.7 fl) by term. This is not due to an exaggerated response in a few women; the distribution of mean cell volumes at term in 153 women not given iron and 147 women given iron throughout pregnancy are shown in Figure 1–1. These values were determined on a Coulter counter, and the range of normal values quoted by the makers of that machine is shown at the top of the figure. Thus the distribution of red cell volumes in those given iron therapy shows a shift to the right. The aggregated effect of the normal red cell count and the increased mean cell volume by term in pregnant women given iron is to return their hemoglobin and hematocrit values to almost prepregnancy levels.

ERYTHROCYTE SEDIMENTATION RATE

Blood from nonpregnant women usually has an ESR of 20 mm per hour or less if whole blood is used and 10 mm or less if the sample is citrated. During pregnancy, the mean ESR is 78 mm with a range of 44 to 114 mm for whole blood and 56 mm with a range of 30 to 98 mm for citrated blood. The reason for this is not clear; if the rise in the ESR is caused by clumping of red cells, the pregnancy effect may be attributed to the increased levels of plasma fibrinogen and globulin. Whatever the origin of this effect, the ESR can be of little diagnostic value during pregnancy.

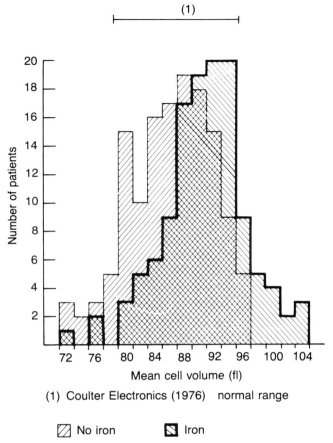

Fig. 1-1. *Distribution of mean cell volume in normal pregnant women at term with and without iron supplementation.*

ERYTHROCYTE FRAGILITY

Because it is expressed in terms of the strength of a sodium chloride solution that causes 50% of the cells placed into it to undergo hemolysis, erythrocyte fragility would be more correctly described as erythrocyte osmotic resistance. For the erythrocytes of nonpregnant women, such a solution would contain 0.435 g/100 ml, but by the last trimester of pregnancy, 0.460 g/100 ml would be required. In other words, the cells must take in much less water before they hemolyze and are therefore more "fragile." The reason for this is probably that the decreased concentration of plasma proteins during pregnancy reduces plasma colloid osmotic pressure; hence, all red cells are slightly more spherical and more prone to "burst."

WHITE CELL COUNT

The total white cell count increases during normal pregnancy, from a prepregnancy mean value of $5.64 \times 10^3/\mu l$ (SD $\pm$ 1.01) to $6.89 \times 10^3/\mu l$ by the end of the first trimester and $10.24 \times 10^3/\mu l$ ($\pm$ 3.39) by 36 weeks. During the immediate puerperium, the white cell count increases still further, and counts of $15 \times 10^3/\mu l$ are not unusual. Such counts, together with a sometimes markedly elevated ESR, could lead the unwary to an incorrect diagnosis of infection. Even as late as 6 weeks postpartum the average count can be $7.27 \times 10^3/\mu l$ ($\pm$ 2.38).

The elevated white cell count is largely a consequence of the increase in the number of neutrophils while there is little change in the number of eosinophils and lymphocytes. Recently, modern electronic counters have enabled accurate platelet counts to be made, and our preliminary serial studies throughout pregnancy suggest that there is a small decrease from a prepregnancy value of about $300 \times 10^3/\mu l$ to $240 \times 10^3/\mu l$ by term, but that women vary widely in this parameter.

SERUM IRON

While requests for determinations of serum iron levels are part of the average daily workload in many biochemistry laboratories, surprisingly little is known about the factors controlling the circulating levels. Wide variations in concentration occur not only between nonpregnant women, but also in the same woman at different times, depending on the season and probably even the time of day. Thus, the usually quoted normal range of 60 to 150 $\mu g/dl$ (11 to 27 $\mu mol/liter$) must be interpreted with caution. Low values can be found even when there are large stores of iron in the marrow.

During normal pregnancy, values usually decrease by 30% to 40%. Routine iron supplementation usually modifies, but does not prevent, this decrease, suggesting that the change is an adaptation to pregnancy rather than an indication of iron insufficiency. This concept is further supported by the fact that serum iron concentrations decrease in the pregnant meat-eating dog—an animal in whom iron insufficiency is unlikely.

SERUM TRANSFERRIN

The concentration of the β_1-globulin transferrin is increased during pregnancy, as are the concentrations of ceruloplasmin and some other carrier proteins. The values in nonpregnant women normally range from 1.2 to 2 g/liter, but have increased by 100% or more by the end of the second trimester. Total iron-binding capacity increases markedly as a consequence of these changes; in nonpregnant women the range is about 250 to 400 $\mu g/dl$ (45 to 72 $\mu mol/liter$), but values around 500 μg/dl (90 μmol/liter) are recorded during the second trimester. While this increase can be reduced somewhat by iron supplementation, the level cannot be returned to the prepregnancy level. This, together with the fact that the total iron-binding capacity increases in women taking combined oral contraceptive agents, suggests that the increased serum transferrin concentration observed in pregnancy may be a response to the increased circulating levels of estrogens.

SERUM FERRITIN

Ferritin, a high molecular weight glycoprotein that is present in most tissues, is the storage compound for tissue iron. It has a life of only a few days and is constantly being replenished. All the ferritin-containing tissues contribute to the plasma ferritin, but the plasma ferritin differs slightly from that in tissues because it is only partially glycosylated and relatively free of iron. It is believed that the amount of ferritin in the circulation is in equilibrium with total body iron stores and, hence, can be used as an index of iron status. In nonpregnant women, a serum concentration of 1 μg/liter is said to be equivalent to 140 μg stored iron per kilogram body weight and values of less than 10 μg/liter would be considered indicative of an iron deficiency.

Ferritin concentrations decrease during normal pregnancy, whether or not iron supplementation is given. In one serial study of 45 pregnant women, 24 women did not receive any supplementation, while the 21 remaining women were given 325 mg ferrous sulfate with 350 μg folic acid daily. In both groups, the serum ferritin level decreased progressively to term, although the mean levels were lower in the unsupplemented group (Fig. 1–2). Indeed, if a level of 10 μg/liter were considered an indication of iron deficiency, many of the women in both groups were iron-deficient. Within 24 hours of delivery, serum ferritin concentrations had increased markedly in both groups of women, suggesting that some pregnancy influence suppresses circulating ferritin levels in a manner unrelated to iron status.

Cord blood ferritin concentrations are substantially greater than maternal levels, and it seems unlikely that the fetal component reaches the mother. In normal pregnancy, there is little relationship between fetal and maternal ferritin concentrations at term. Some investigators believe, however, that cord blood values are relatively lower in babies born to iron-deficient mothers.

RED CELL PROTOPORPHYRIN

Free protoporphyrin in the erythrocytes increases by a small amount during normal pregnancy; in one series, the values in women who were not given iron supplements increased from an average of 0.25 mg/liter erythrocytes to about 0.35

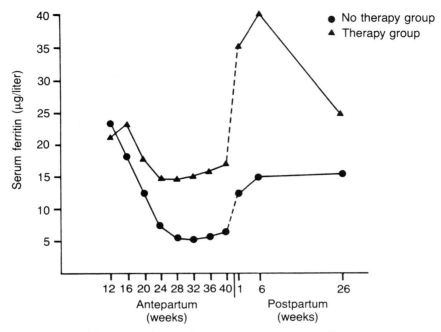

Fig. 1-2. *Effect of hematinic therapy during pregnancy on serum iron.*

mg/liter, but there was a wide range of values among the individuals. This physiologic adjustment is again in the direction of iron deficiency, in which values between 0.5 and 3 mg/liter may be found. The cause and significance of this change in pregnancy is unknown.

BLOOD GLUCOSE

Although glucose is carried in both the red cells and plasma, it is the glucose in plasma that is available to the tissues and stimulates insulin release and appropriate glucagon feedback control. Capillary blood obtained from the fingers or ear lobes is arterial and has a higher concentration of glucose than does blood obtained by venipuncture. Thus published reports ought to state clearly how the blood sample was obtained and whether the determinations were made on whole blood or plasma.

As glucose is evenly distributed through the water phase of plasma and red cells, a knowledge of the water content of erythrocytes and plasma, as well as the hematocrit, makes it possible to extrapolate plasma glucose concentrations from whole blood values. For example, if the hematocrit is 34%, if the water content of red cells is 65%, and if the water content of plasma is 93%, the water space available to glucose is 83.5% in whole blood and 93% in plasma. Hence, plasma concentrations will be higher than whole blood values by 93:83.5 or 1.114 times.

Fasting values have occasionally been reported to be unaffected by pregnancy, but the weight of published evidence suggests a slight decrease. Interestingly, a decrease of 8 to 10 mg/dl occurs within the first trimester with little change thereafter. This does not support the theory that this reduction is caused by fetal demand. It is also unrelated to any change in the fasting plasma insulin level.

Postprandial glucose concentrations do change progressively as gestation advances. In nonpregnant women, peak values are usually reached approximately 30 minutes after an oral glucose load; in pregnant women at term, approximately 55 minutes after an oral glucose load. The average maximum concentration achieved after a 50-g oral glucose load is about 112 mg/dl in nonpregnant women, but about 122 mg/dl in women who are near term. The whole response curve is more rounded (Fig. 1–3), with the implication that, while fasting values are usually regained within 2 hours in the postprandial phase, blood glucose values are elevated for longer during pregnancy. This makes physiologic sense because glucose crosses the

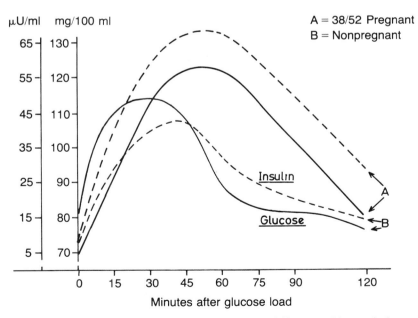

Fig. 1-3. *Mean plasma glucose and insulin concentrations following a 50-g oral glucose load in healthy women at 38 weeks of normal pregnancy and the same women 12 weeks postdelivery (labeled nonpregnant).*

placenta to the fetus by diffusion; hence the maintenance of an increased gradient between mother and fetus facilitates transfer of this vital nutrient to the fetus.

FOLATE

The commonly prescribed pharmacologic preparation known as folic acid does not occur in nature. The vitamin should more correctly be referred to as folate, since dietary intake is usually in the form of folate monoglutamates or polyglutamates and since administered folic acid is reduced in the same way that folate is reduced (i.e., first to dihydrofolic acid and then to tetrahydrofolic acid, the usable form at cellular level). Because it is essential for cell growth, folate requirements are increased during pregnancy; it is needed for the development of the fetus and placenta, as well as for the uterine hypertrophy of the mother.

Circulating plasma folate levels are generally decreased during pregnancy, but there are wide variations not only between women, but also in the same woman at different times, particularly in relation to meals. It is thus impossible to state unequivocally the plasma folate level that indicates a deficiency in a pregnant patient. For example, one study showed that the range in nonpregnant women was 3 to 13 μg/liter, with a mean of 6 μg/liter. The range in pregnant women was 1 to 9 μg/liter with a mean of 3 μg/liter. Thus approximately 50% of all healthy pregnant women appear to have values below the lower normal range.

It has been suggested that red cell folate concentrations may reflect tissue levels more accurately. Again, absolute levels cannot be quoted because of the wide variations among individuals and differences in the laboratory methods used to determine folate concentrations. It is known, however, that concentrations decrease during normal pregnancy. While folate levels in plasma and red cells are reduced in patients with megaloblastic anemia, the overlap of their concentrations with the range found in normal healthy women is so great that a diagnosis of megaloblastic anemia should not be based on blood levels alone.

The mechanism by which folate levels are reduced in women who eat a folate-sufficient diet is not yet understood. While malabsorption of the vitamin from the intestines is possible, there is no good evidence that this is the cause. Urinary excretion is increased by about 8 weeks of gestation, presumably reflecting the increase that occurs in the glomerular filtration rate (GFR) during the first trimester, but this can be only a marginal cause of lower plasma folate levels, if important at all. Folate levels decrease throughout the greater part of pregnancy, while the GFR reaches its maximum value between 12 and 16 weeks.

The excretion of formiminoglutamic acid has been used in the past as a test of folate status. If a loading dose of histidine is given, increased amounts of formiminoglutamic acid are excreted in the urine of a woman who has a folate deficiency. The metabolism of histidine is altered during pregnancy, however, and the excretion of formiminoglutamic acid is normally increased during the first trimester.

Cord blood folate levels are invariably higher than those of the mother. In one remarkable instance, a very ill Nigerian mother had no detectable folate in her blood, yet the fetus had easily detectable levels. The way in which this mechanism of fetal privilege works is unknown. It is more complex than active or facilitated transport from mother to fetus, because the highest levels of all are found in the placenta. In some way, the placenta can accept and store folate, even to the physical disadvantage of the mother. The fetal circulating levels are low compared with those of the placenta, and the gradient between placental and fetal concentration rather than that between maternal and fetal concentration may be the governing influence.

VITAMIN B_{12}

Concentrations of vitamin B_{12} appear to decrease progressively in both red cells and serum during pregnancy. Available data suggest that muscle levels are also reduced. If the concentration is determined by a method yielding a range of 105 to 1,025 ng/liter in nonpregnant women, for example, the corresponding range at term would be 20 to 510 ng/liter, with even lower levels in women having a multiple pregnancy. In addition, cigarette smoking appears to reduce B_{12} levels, and the effect is presumably additive if pregnant women smoke.

There are two B_{12} binding proteins. Transcobalamin I is derived from leukocytes and is increased in myeloproliferative conditions, but not during pregnancy. Transcobalamin II is derived from the liver, and it is this fraction that increases during pregnancy, increasing the body's binding capacity for B_{12}. There appears to be a genetic difference governing these proteins, because West Indian Blacks living in Great Britain who have a slightly smaller dietary B_{12} intake have serum levels about twice those of Europeans, presumably indicating an increased binding capacity.

B_{12} levels may be very low in folate-deficient women and will increase after therapy with folate alone. Therefore, it is necessary to exclude folate deficiency before making a diagnosis of true B_{12} deficiency on blood levels alone.

Cord blood B_{12} levels are higher than maternal levels, but the fetus does not seem to have the same protection it enjoys with respect to folate. The infants of some vegetarian Hindu women who have low serum B_{12} levels are born with subnormal levels, even though their levels are higher than the maternal levels.

ERYTHROPOIETIN

Until recently, the level of erythropoietin could be determined only by bioassay methods, but reliable immunoassay techniques are now available. Although pregnancy data are limited, one serial study has been done of ten women throughout pregnancy; six of the women were studied over their conceptual cycle so that data were obtained literally from the beginning of pregnancy.

The level of erythropoietin increased progressively throughout pregnancy. There was a wide spectrum of individual responses, as shown by the wide standard deviation around the mean values (Fig. 1–4); nevertheless, each woman showed a progressive elevation in her erythropoietin level (Fig. 1–5). This finding is somewhat paradoxical. The hormone increases steadily, as does total red cell mass, which could be expected; however, the normal stimulus for erythropoietin production is tissue hypoxemia, and this would be unusual during pregnancy. Not only is the pregnant woman's oxygen-carrying capacity improved in terms of the increase in total circulating hemoglobin, but also the arteriovenous oxygen difference at the heart is reduced (i.e., better oxygenated blood is returned to the heart). Hence, the stimulus for the sustained release of erythropoietin remains an enigma, again illustrating that the mother's homeostatic status is completely altered during pregnancy.

The limited data available suggest that cord blood erythropoietin concentrations are higher than maternal concentrations when paired samples are examined. At full term, however, the mean cord blood value is not different from the mean maternal value. Sheep and goat studies suggest that fetal erythropoietin cannot

Fig. 1-4. *Mean serum erythropoietin concentrations (± 1 SD) throughout pregnancy. Values are expressed in terms of concentrations above a low erythropoietin serum pool value (LESP).*

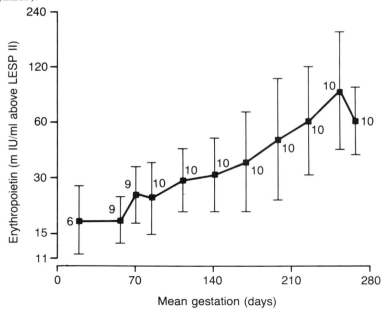

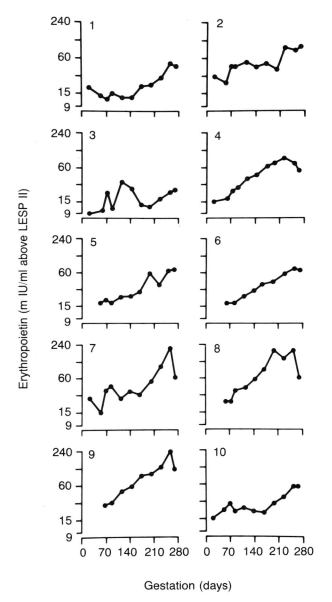

Fig. 1-5. *Serial erythropoietin concentrations for the 10 individual patients whose mean values are shown in Figure 1–4.*

cross the placenta. The same is probably true in humans, but no data are available to confirm this at the present time.

ANEMIA

In everyday practice, the diagnosis of iron deficiency anemia is based on the finding of a low hemoglobin concentration. But what is "low"? Red cell mass goes up by 20% or more during pregnancy, but plasma volume increases by 30% to 50%; hence, when expressed as a concentration, the hemoglobin value must go down. If a nonpregnant woman has a hemoglobin of 13 g/dl and a total blood volume of 3,500 ml, for example, she has 455 g total circulating hemoglobin. During a subsequent pregnancy, her hemoglobin may decrease to 9.5 g/dl and her blood volume increase to 5,000 ml; this is equivalent to a total circulating hemoglobin of 475 g. Is she anemic?

During normal pregnancy, serum iron concentrations decrease markedly, while the transferrin concentration increases; inevitably, iron-binding capacity increases. Red cell protoporphyrin increases a little, and serum ferritin decreases. Thus, virtually all standard laboratory indices favor a diagnosis of iron insufficiency. On the other hand, women who have hypertensive complications of pregnancy and some women whose fetus displays intrauterine growth retardation have a reduction in their plasma volume. As a consequence, their hemoglobin concentration is often in the "normal" range—but are they less iron-deficient?

Only true iron deficiency and thalassemia cause microcythemia. Because the mean cell volume does not change during normal pregnancy in women who do not take iron, it is probably the best single indicator of iron status. A mean cell volume of 82 μm^3 or more is unlikely to be associated with true iron deficiency. The life span of a red cell is 120 days, however, so that it is some time before sufficient small red cells are present in the circulation to affect the mean cell volume. Hence, a progressive decrease in mean cell volume with an associated decrease in hemoglobin concentration deserves attention.

Iron insufficiency that requires therapy is bound to occur in some pregnant women. Indeed, some general populations show evidence of iron insufficiency, and pregnancy can only aggravate such an insufficiency. Clearly, pregnant women require more thoughtful consideration of laboratory findings than a mere judgment in terms of "normal" standards. This is true of virtually every major physiologic system.

BLOOD VISCOSITY

It can be argued that the increase in the volume of plasma relative to that of the contained cells makes blood less viscid, thus improving its flow along capillary vessels, reducing the work required of the heart, and helping to keep blood pressure down as cardiac output increases. The diameters of many capillary vessels are smaller than the diameter of normal red cells; flow in such vessels is a function of the flexibility of red cells and their ability to elongate and adapt their shape to travel down such capillaries. While laboratory measurements of whole blood viscosity may not reflect the circumstances inside a blood vessel, it has been reported that, relative to distilled water, whole blood viscosity decreases from 4.61 in nonpregnant women to 4.2 during early pregnancy and 3.84 by about 28 weeks of gestation.

The possible effects on small vessel flow of returning the hematocrit to near nonpregnancy levels and increasing the volume of individual red cells by iron supplementation must at least be considered. In otherwise normal healthy pregnant women who are having uncomplicated pregnancies, for example, there is an inverse relationship between maternal hemoglobin concentration in late pregnancy and infant birthweight.

Biochemical and General Composition of Serum and Plasma

OSMOLALITY

Total osmolality decreases remarkably during the first trimester from an average nonpregnancy value of 291 to 281 mosm/kg by 12 weeks of gestation (when determined as a depression of the freezing point). From 12 weeks of gestation to term, there is little further change.

Plasma osmolality is rigidly controlled in healthy people. Drinking a liter of water normally reduces plasma osmolality by approximately 10 mosm/kg, provoking a diuresis. Within 2 hours, the majority of this fluid load has been passed as urine and total osmolality returns to the starting level. If a pregnant woman is given a liter of water to drink, her plasma osmolality also decreases by 10 mosm/kg to a new low of about 270 mosm/kg; she has an even more efficient diuresis, however, and she returns to her "normal" value of about 280 mosm/kg within 60 to 90 minutes.

Under these circumstances, it may seem curious that pregnant women are not in a permanent state of diabetes insipidus. For a short time, they may experience a mild increase in urine excretion—the so-called frequency of micturition that occurs in early pregnancy. Pregnant women not only tolerate this lowered osmolality, however, but also guard their osmolality as keenly as do their nonpregnant counterparts. Thus it must be accepted that the new value is a desirable physiologic adjustment to pregnancy. The implication is that, during pregnancy, the osmoreceptors in the hypothalamus are re-set to accept this new homeostatic level.

The reason for the osmolality change is not fully understood. It is a measure of the total number of dissolved particles in a solution. In the case of plasma, this implies all substances (e.g., urea, creatinine, and glucose), but sodium and chloride predominate. The theoretical reduction in osmolality that should occur can be calculated from the known changes in the various solute concentrations and agrees closely with the measured drop of about 10 mosm/kg.

Colloid osmotic pressure is expressed in centimeters of water at 37°C. Values are between 37 and 38 cm in a nonpregnant woman and decrease to approximately 30 to 31 cm by about 24 weeks of gestation, closely resembling the decrease in plasma albumin concentration. As albumin is the smallest of the plasma proteins, it seems reasonable to infer that this is the causative factor, but the reason for a change in colloid osmotic pressure is again obscure. Theoretically, such a change should cause water to leave the vascular compartment for the tissues, resulting in edema. That edema does occur is well-known; the maximum decrease in colloid osmotic pressure has occurred by about 20 weeks, however, while clinically obvious edema usually manifests itself during the third trimester. It can be speculated that a blood pressure decrease during the middle trimester is the balancing factor, because it is blood pressure (or, more accurately, venous pressure) that tends to drive fluid from the vascular space while colloid attraction maintains it there. Hence, the reduced osmotic attraction may be offset by the reduced venous pressure during the first half of pregnancy; later, as blood pressure increases, water tends to leave the vascular space and edema becomes more evident.

ELECTROLYTES

The **sodium** level decreases from an average nonpregnancy concentration of 140 mEq/liter to 137 mEq/liter by 12 weeks, a value that is maintained to term with only minor fluctuations within an individual from occasion to occasion. It is often suggested that aldosterone is a major influence on sodium balance, and it is true that disturbances of aldosterone secretion do affect sodium balance. However, if an average GFR is about 100 ml/min and if sodium concentration is 140 mEq/liter, then 140 mEq is filtered every 10 minutes; this amounts to more than 20,000 mEq per day, of which only about 200 mEq or 1% is excreted. If the sodium concentration decreases during pregnancy to about 137 mEq/liter, but the GFR increases to about 150 ml/min, then 30,000 mEq is filtered each day. The fact that there is little increase in the urinary excretion per 24 hours shows that the reabsorptive capacity of the renal tubules is sufficient to cope with these large increases in filtered load. Indeed, it is the reabsorption of this extra sodium that is the major renal adaptation of pregnancy. Aldosterone probably acts as a "fine tuner" of the system and facilitates the reabsorption of sodium from more distal portions of the tubule if the proximal tubular sites are transiently overcome.

Potassium decreases from a nonpregnancy average of 3.9 mEq/liter to approximately 3.6 mEq/liter by 12 weeks. While this may not seem particularly impressive, the decrease in potassium is about 8%, while that in sodium is about 2%. Concentrations may increase slightly toward term.

Calcium changes bring a further problem for consideration: the effect of protein binding. Many factors are transported by blood in both a free and a bound state. Their biologic effect is caused by the free fraction. When this is inactivated or metabolized, more is released from the binding protein so that the equilibrium between the free and bound fractions is maintained. Thus, the concept of concentration as a biologically useful value must embrace not only increases in plasma volume, but also the interrelated factors, such as changes in total protein concentration, the presence of specific binding proteins for various compounds, and the possible effects of competitors for the same binding sites. Usually, assays detect only total concentrations, but advances in laboratory techniques are making it possible to obtain more specific data.

Total calcium concentrations decrease during pregnancy to term values about 10% below the average nonpregnancy level: 10.2 mg/dl (2.5 mmol/liter) to approximately 9.2 mg/dl (2.3 mmol/liter). This is consistent with the decrease in plasma albumin concentration. More recent work has suggested that a smaller, but significant decrease in serum ionic calcium concentrations occurs between the first and third trimesters.

With the use of a nonradioactive tracer (calcium 48), it has been shown that calcium absorption increases during the early weeks of pregnancy and has doubled by 24 weeks of gestation. Urinary calcium excretion also increases, but even after this "wastage," the calcium retained is more than enough to meet the needs of both the mother and her developing fetus. Although early studies tended to indicate increased mobilization of calcium from the maternal skeleton, implying a one-way transfer or "loss," it now seems that there is an increase in the total calcium turnover of the mother's exchangeable bone calcium and that fetal needs are met without any net loss from the maternal skeleton in a normally nourished woman. Calcium absorption from the upper part of the small intestine is dependent on the presence of $1,25(OH)_2$-cholecalciferol, while renal reabsorption is governed by parathyroid hormone (PTH).

Magnesium decreases, too, and recent data suggest that this may be evident soon after conception. Ten patients followed longitudinally from preconception to postdelivery had an average prepregnancy value of 2.1 ± 0.15 mg/dl (0.87 ± 0.06 mmol/liter) ($n = 31$), decreasing to 1.6 ± 0.2 mg/dl (0.67 ± 0.08 mmol/liter) ($n = 10$) at 32 weeks. (Each patient had been studied on more than one occasion prior to pregnancy.) A small increase in concentration probably occurs between 32 weeks and term (Fig. 1–6). Absorption of magnesium from the gut and renal reabsorption is under the control of PTH. Iron supplementation does not appear to affect absorption.

Zinc decreases from an average prepregnancy value of 883 ± 92 mg/liter (13.5 ± 1.4 mmol/liter) ($n = 31$) to a nadir of 635 ± 56 mg/liter (9.71 ± 0.86 mmol/liter) at 36 weeks (Fig. 1–6). As with magnesium, a small increase occurs thereafter to term. If the increase in plasma volume is taken into account, however, the total amount of circulating zinc remains virtually unchanged. Indeed, the initial "decrease" can be accounted for by the "reduced" amount of circulating albumin.

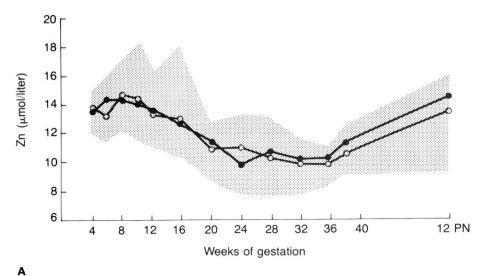

A

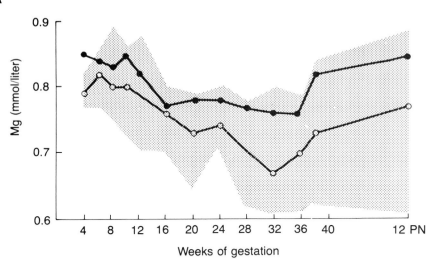

B

Fig. 1-6. *Changes in serum concentrations of zinc (**A**) and magnesium (**B**) in 10 healthy women who did not take iron supplementation during pregnancy (open circles) and 10 women who did take regular supplementation during pregnancy (closed circles). Range in each case is shown as stippled area.*

In reality, the *total* amount of circulating albumin is unchanged, so the available binding capacity of the major carrier protein is also unchanged. Time and again, it is clear that reduced concentrations of any particular substance do not necessarily imply a reduction in the total amount of the substance that is in the circulation and hence available to the tissues and fetus.

Concentrations of **copper** increase from average prepregnancy values of 1.14 mg/liter (18 μmol/liter) to 2.03 mg/liter (32 μmol/liter) by term. As the fetal liver contains about ten times the amount of copper found in the adult liver on an equivalent weight basis, it has been postulated that maternal copper levels increase in response to fetal demand. Maternal ceruloplasmin, the specific copper-binding protein, increases in concentration during pregnancy, however, as do many of the binding proteins. Copper levels may increase in response to this improved binding capacity.

While there is little, if any, change in circulating **chloride** levels during pregnancy, bicarbonate concentrations decrease by approximately 4 mEq/liter to values between 18 and 22 mEq/liter. This may be an example of the many physiologic checks and balances that are required for one important physiologic adaptation. The following argument is made to fit the observed facts logically; it should be regarded as illustrative rather than "fact."

Because the developing fetus must be able to off-load its **bicarbonate**, maternal P_{CO_2} decreases from the prepregnancy average of 39 mm Hg to approximately 31 mm Hg. A persistent lowering of the P_{CO_2} would lead to maternal alkalosis, yet pH is maintained. Therefore, there must be a compensatory loss of bicarbonate via the kidneys to account for the decreased sodium concentrations and, in turn, the reduction in total osmolality. As pregnant women do not develop diabetes insipidus, the osmoreceptors must be reset, and so on. Hence, in order to allow the fetus to off-load its CO_2, the mother undergoes a cascade of marked physiologic adaptations.

Phosphate concentrations in serum and urine change little, if at all, throughout pregnancy. While vitamin D facilitates phosphate absorption from the gut, much can be absorbed even without the vitamin. Unlike calcium, phosphate occurs intracellularly in large amounts, and circulating levels are regulated by renal filtration and absorption.

PROTEINS

Total protein concentrations decrease by about 10 g/liter during pregnancy. The major change occurs during the first trimester, beginning by about the fourth week of gestation, dated from the first day of the last menstrual period (i.e., from about 2 weeks postimplantation). The effect is due largely to the decrease in the concentration of albumin, which exactly parallels the change in total protein, decreasing from about 47 to 36 g/liter. If the average nonpregnancy plasma volume is 2,300 ml and if the albumin concentration is 47 g/liter, there is 108 g albumin circulating; at a pregnancy volume of about 3,600 ml, the reduced albumin concentration of 36 g/liter still means a total of 129.6 g albumin is in the vascular space.

The implications for protein production are interesting. The major decrease in **albumin** concentrations has occurred by the end of the first trimester, although there is a further gradual decrease to approximately 24 weeks. Plasma volume, on the other hand, shows no change in the first trimester, but increases progressively thereafter to approximately 36 weeks. There must be a decrease in the production of albumin during the first 12 weeks, but an increase in production thereafter to maintain concentrations in the face of an increasing blood volume. The alternative, an alteration in the metabolic clearance of protein, seems less likely.

The term **globulin** embraces a family of globulins, each of which has its characteristic changes during pregnancy. The overall concentration of globulins increases slightly, although the concentration of some individual globulins decreases. For example, the concentrations of the α_1-globulin and α_2-globulin fractions increase (each by about 1 g/liter), and there is a larger increase in the β-globulin fraction (about 2 to 3 g/liter). The concentrations of the γ-globulins decrease slightly, however. There is some disagreement about the relative changes of the different γ-globulins, but it seems likely that the γ-G fraction decreases while the γ-A and γ-M fractions remain unchanged or perhaps increase slightly. The specific thyroxine-binding globulin doubles in concentration.

Maternal α-fetoprotein is an α_1-glycoprotein made in the fetal liver and yolk sac. At 12 to 14 weeks of gestation, it comprises approximately one-third of the total plasma proteins in the fetus, but declines to approximately 1% at term. Its physiologic significance as a plasma protein in the fetus distinct from albumin is unknown, but the fact that its amino acid sequences have many similarities to those of albumin suggest a common ancestral source for these substances. The much lower maternal levels of α-fetoprotein derive from the fetus and increase progressively toward term. Absolute values reported vary from center to center, depending on the methods and standards used, but concentrations usually range between 100 and 550 μg/liter at term. Women who have had an intrauterine death may have levels in excess of 8,000 μg/liter, however.

Pregnancy-specific proteins are known by a variety of names. Of the 20 or so described so far, three have evoked clinical interest: Schwangerschafts protein 1 (SP1), pregnancy-associated plasma protein A (PAPP-A), and placental protein 5 (PP5). Because SP1, which may be two proteins (SP1α and SP1β), appears in the circulation as early as does human chorionic gonadotropin (hCG), an immunoassay for its detection has been suggested as a pregnancy test. Its function, if any, awaits clarification, however. PAPP-A and PP5 may have some local action to prevent fibrinolysis at the placenta, but few facts are yet established. Indeed, elucidation of the formation and function of these placental proteins will be one of the growing edges of future obstetric research.

ENZYMES

The family of substances categorized by the word *enzyme* is extremely large. Data concerned with changes during pregnancy are available on the following enzymes.

Serum concentrations of **lactate dehydrogenase, isocitrate dehydrogenase, and α-hydroxybutyrate dehydrogenase** appear to be unaffected by pregnancy, but the data available are generally from cross-sectional studies; longitudinal studies may reveal small increases toward term within individuals. Concentrations of all three enzymes appear to increase during labor.

17β-Hydroxysteroid oxidoreductase, which is formed in the placenta, is detectable by about the tenth week of gestation. Its level increases tenfold by term. It appears to catalyze the oxidation–reduction of estrone and estradiol.

Monoamine oxidase levels appear to be unchanged during pregnancy, although the evidence is indirect. This enzyme degrades 5-hydroxytryptamine (5-HT), also known as serotonin, to its metabolite 5-hydroxyindoleacetic acid (5-HIAA), which is excreted in the urine. A dose of 5-HT given to pregnant women yields the same excretion of 5-HIAA as in nonpregnant women.

Diamine oxidase (or histaminase) increases in concentration about tenfold by term, from approximately 0.1 IU/liter to 1 IU/liter. Unfortunately, even though enzyme assays are usually pH- and temperature-dependent, these factors are rarely mentioned in published reports. The pH is of particular interest in regard to diamine oxidase, because assays are sometimes performed at pH 7.4 and the optimum activity of this enzyme is at pH 6.9.

Ceruloplasmin activity in a pregnant woman is almost twice that in a nonpregnant woman. This copper-containing oxidase may act to counter the possibly toxic side effects of the increasing serotonin levels that occur during normal pregnancy. It may also be responsible for the increase in serum copper described earlier.

Glutamic-oxalacetic transaminase (GOT) and **glutamic-pyruvic transaminase** (GPT) serum levels appear to be unaffected by pregnancy, but may increase during labor. GOT levels of 9.3 ± 5.6 IU/liter have been reported in laboring women, compared to late pregnancy values of 6.2 ± 3.5 IU/liter; these values for GPT are 7.0 ± 3.9 IU/liter and 5.4 ± 2.8 IU/liter, respectively. Of interest, though as yet without explanation, is the observation that concentrations in excess of 80 IU/liter for GOT and 58 IU/liter for GPT have been reported in some women with a hydatidiform mole.

Creatine kinase levels at term appear to be about the same as levels in normal, nonpregnant women (i.e., approximately 28 IU/liter). During the first half of pregnancy, however, serum levels appear to be reduced (21 IU/liter) and increase thereafter in much the same way as uric acid values increase. This could be of some importance for women who wish to be counseled during early pregnancy about the possibility that their offspring may have Duchenne muscular dystrophy.

Lipase, more fully lipoprotein lipase, activity in plasma appears to be markedly reduced during pregnancy, from values of about 40 ± 5 IU/liter to about 16 ± 6 IU/liter. The reason for this is uncertain, but it is presumably related to the increased circulating lipid concentrations during pregnancy.

Pseudocholinesterase, found principally in plasma, splits virtually any choline ester, not just acetylcholine. Cholinesterase is found mainly in tissues and has the greater affinity for acetylcholine. Levels of pseudocholinesterase in pregnancy are probably some 20% to 40% below nonpregnancy values, which could be of some importance to anesthetists if they use succinylcholine as a muscle relaxant during surgery on pregnant women; the action of this drug may be undesirably prolonged.

Alkaline phosphatase was named because "it" hydrolyzes monoesters of orthophosphoric acid at an alkaline pH. In reality, the term denotes a family of isoenzymes that have a genetically determined pattern within an individual. The serum activity of alkaline phosphatase increases threefold to fivefold during pregnancy; some change is discernible by approximately 20 weeks of gestation. This increase is due almost exclusively to a fraction that is formed in the placenta and can be easily identified because it is still stable after heating to 65°C. It forms 40 to 60% of circulating serum alkaline phosphatase at term, making the diagnosis of liver disease based on this enzyme more difficult. Despite considerable research, alkaline phosphatase appears to have little value as an indicator of placental function.

Acid phosphatase activity in serum does not increase at all during pregnancy. Values of 1.3 ± 0.1, 1.5 ± 0.2, and 1.7 ± 0.3 IU/liter are found during the first, second, and third trimesters, respectively, compared to a nonpregnancy level of 1.4 ± 0.15 IU/liter.

α-**Amylase** (diastase) activity does not appear to be affected by pregnancy. Values of 2,370 ± 700 IU/liter are recorded at term, compared to nonpregnancy values of 2,310 ± 660 IU/liter. This does not exclude the possibility that the concentration decreases during the first half of pregnancy and returns to "normal" during the second half, much as the levels of creatine kinase and uric acid do; however, data are lacking.

The **cystine and leucine aminopeptidases** both increase in concentration during pregnancy because the placenta produces them. Both split peptide chains and therefore help in the destruction of polypeptide hormones. Cystine aminopeptidase is the "oxytocinase" that has been described and, in humans, is probably responsible for the rapid inactivation of the antidiuretic hormone arginine vasopressin.

LIPIDS

Generally, the concentrations of serum lipids increase progressively throughout pregnancy. As with the proteins, however, there are different changes in the various fractions. Lipids are transported in the blood as lipoproteins. Until relatively recent times, they were classified as α- and β-lipoproteins, the α fraction moving with α-globulin and the β fraction moving with the β-globulins on electrophoresis. More recently, they have been classified according to their density based on ultracentrifugation: very low density lipoproteins (VLDL), low density lipoproteins (LDL), and high density lipoproteins (HDL).

Triglyceride levels increase progressively throughout pregnancy from about 1 g/liter to 2 or 3 g/liter by term. Levels of VLDL and LDL increase about fourfold, which is proportionally similar to the increase in the levels of cholesterol and the phospholipids; levels of LDL and HDL triglycerides increase much more than those of the other two lipid groups.

Cholesterol doubles from 1 g/liter at the end of the first trimester to approximately 2 g/liter by 34 weeks of gestation; like uric acid and creatine kinase, however, cholesterol decreases in concentration during the early weeks of pregnancy. It is difficult to explain these changes. Diet has little effect, as vegetarians show the same increasing cholesterol concentrations as do those who eat meat and eggs. If a diet is deliberately selected to be low in saturated fats and high in polyunsaturated fats, serum cholesterol levels decrease in nonpregnant women, but such a diet has no influence at all on the usual changes in pregnant women. Paradoxically, the IV administration of glucose and insulin normally reduces the level of circulating cholesterol, but increases it during pregnancy. Yet, as far as can be determined, pregnancy has no effect on cholesterol metabolism or the rate of cholesterol synthesis. Indeed, the fact that the level of HDL triglyceride increases without a reduction in the level of HDL cholesterol distinguishes normal pregnancy physiology from hyperlipoproteinemias.

Phospholipids increase their overall serum concentration from about 2.5 to 4 g/liter during pregnancy, but the VLDL fraction increases proportionally more than the LDL and HDL fractions increase. In biochemical terms, the cephalins increase about threefold, the lecithins and sphingomyelins increase about twofold, but the lysolecithins decrease somewhat. The fatty acid composition of the phospholipids may also change with a rise in palmitic and oleic acids and fall in linoleic and arachidonic acids.

Nonesterified fatty acids are sometimes referred to as "free" fatty acids. Because there is no basal or "fasted" status when a patient's fatty acid concentrations can be expected to be uniform from occasion to occasion, as there is with glucose, changes that may result from pregnancy are difficult to identify. Serum levels are affected by such factors as the duration of fasting, emotional stress, the effect of the venipuncture to obtain the sample, and cigarette smoking. Despite all these variables, there is surprising unanimity among published reports that nonesterified fatty acid values are considerably increased during the last trimester. Methodologic differences, as well as all the variables, make it impossible to give sensible means or ranges for the concentrations, however.

NONPROTEIN NITROGEN

Urea concentration is a commonly requested laboratory measurement, yet there is little uniformity of reporting. Some laboratories return serum levels, while others return plasma or even whole blood values. Urea nitrogen values, which are approximately half of urea values, are sometimes reported. In the following discussions, serum concentrations are given.

From a mean nonpregnancy value of 25.4 ± 4.74 mg/dl (4.24 ± 0.79 mmol/liter), serum urea concentrations decrease to 18.9 ± 3.9 mg/dl (3.16 ± 0.66 mmol/liter) by 12 weeks; a further progressive, but smaller, decrease occurs to 32 weeks, when values average 15.3 ± 3.4 mg/dl (2.55 ± 0.56 mmol/liter). Thereafter, there is a small increase, with values at 38 weeks being 17.4 ± 3.8 mg/dl (2.90 ± 0.64 mmol/liter; Table 1–7; Fig. 1–7). This pronounced decrease has usually been attributed to an increased renal clearance of urea, but these data show that serum concentrations have decreased by 4 to 6 weeks of gestation when renal clearance may not have begun to increase; it must be considered that a change in protein metabolism occurs (i.e., the rate of protein breakdown may decrease early in pregnancy).

Changes in serum **creatinine** concentrations appear to parallel those of urea. The mean value at 12 weeks of gestation is 0.68 mg/dl (60.53 μmol/liter), compared to the nonpregnancy average of 0.89 mg/dl (78.76 μmol/liter). A further slow decrease occurs with values reaching a nadir at 32 weeks and increasing slightly toward term (Table 1–7).

The decrease in serum urea by 12 weeks is about 26%; the decrease in serum creatinine is about 23%. As both solutes are decreased to approximately the same proportional extent, they could be reflecting a change in renal function (i.e., increased clearance). Urine creatinine concentration, which is less susceptible to dietary influences, remains relatively constant throughout pregnancy (Table 1–7), however. As there is little change in the volume of urine passed per day, the total

Table 1-7. *Serum urea, serum creatinine, and urine creatinine concentrations (mg/dl) throughout pregnancy*

Weeks of Gestation	Number of Observations	Serum Urea	Serum Creatinine	Urine Creatinine
4	16	22.4 ± 4.5	0.85 ± 0.11	0.090 ± 0.016
6	26	21.8 ± 4.4	0.79 ± 0.10	0.101 ± 0.031
8	30	20.8 ± 4.9	0.74 ± 0.09	0.098 ± 0.028 *
10	31	19.1 ± 4.4	0.71 ± 0.09	0.096 ± 0.029
12	34	19.0 ± 4.0	0.68 ± 0.08	0.090 ± 0.023 †
16	37	18.1 ± 4.4	0.69 ± 0.08	0.091 ± 0.025
20	35	17.6 ± 3.5	0.67 ± 0.10	0.089 ± 0.030
24	37	17.1 ± 3.2	0.66 ± 0.10	0.090 ± 0.025
28	36	16.6 ± 3.4	0.66 ± 0.09	0.085 ± 0.022 ‡
32	36	15.3 ± 3.4	0.66 ± 0.08	0.089 ± 0.035
36	36	16.6 ± 3.5	0.70 ± 0.08	0.091 ± 0.035
38	32	17.4 ± 3.8	0.73 ± 0.10	0.090 ± 0.030

* Only 20 observations
† Only 33 observations
‡ Only 35 observations

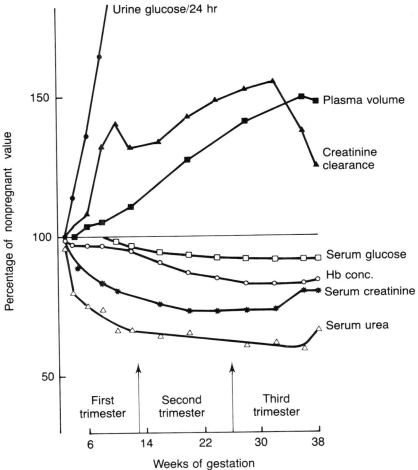

Fig. 1-7. *Values associated with physiologic changes occurring throughout pregnancy expressed as a proportion of nonpregnant values (100%). Data are from a longitudinal study of healthy women who yielded their own nonpregnant control values.*

excretion of creatinine per 24 hours is also relatively unchanged. More data are required to clarify whether changes in serum solute concentrations reflect altered renal function, a change in maternal metabolism, or a combination of both.

Amino acid concentrations change in a complex and little understood way. No easily discernible patterns appear when the individual amino acids are grouped according to their biochemical characteristics (e.g., basic or acidic). Most studies have shown an overall decrease in the total amino acid concentration of maternal blood during pregnancy, but there are so many differences in the laboratory methods used that it would be misleading to report specific values. To date, only one study has included serial values on the same women throughout pregnancy (Table 1–8).

Table 1-8. *Plasma amino acids (μmol/liter) throughout pregnancy in 10 healthy women having uncomplicated pregnancies*

Amino Acid	Under 20 Weeks	20–29 Weeks	30 Weeks and over	8 Weeks Postpartum
Alanine	295 ± 56	338 ± 69	341 ± 89	382 ± 128
Arginine	80 ± 24	68 ± 31	59 ± 23	75 ± 33
Asparagine	28 ± 9	28 ± 13	27 ± 13	32 ± 23
Cystine	22 ± 9	37 ± 24	24 ± 11	33 ± 21
Glutamic acid	145 ± 56	148 ± 79	167 ± 64	162 ± 71
Glycine	161 ± 37	154 ± 37	132 ± 44	246 ± 105
Histidine	92 ± 22	92 ± 11	93 ± 17	92 ± 34
Isoleucine	58 ± 19	50 ± 15	49 ± 11	56 ± 23
Leucine	100 ± 27	99 ± 20	85 ± 18	105 ± 46
Lysine	163 ± 41	170 ± 31	152 ± 26	212 ± 99
Methionine	12 ± 8	13 ± 7	12 ± 5	18 ± 15
Ornithine	46 ± 10	53 ± 13	46 ± 15	93 ± 43
Phenylalanine	54 ± 18	56 ± 13	50 ± 9	61 ± 24
Proline	150 ± 58	151 ± 62	167 ± 51	251 ± 88
Serine	135 ± 50	143 ± 62	118 ± 44	169 ± 73
Taurine	80 ± 34	75 ± 26	62 ± 15	104 ± 69
Threonine	295 ± 46	378 ± 75	354 ± 106	400 ± 118
Tyrosine	47 ± 18	42 ± 6	45 ± 6	68 ± 31
Valine	186 ± 45	178 ± 41	156 ± 33	204 ± 93

Compared with nonpregnancy levels, there are pronounced decreases in the concentrations of ornithine, glycine, taurine, and proline during pregnancy, but the reason for these decreases remains an enigma. Red cell values of the amino acids increase during pregnancy, presumably indicating their enhanced tissue uptake by the mother; glutamic acid is the exception. Glutamic acid is also unusual in that its plasma level tends to increase between 10 weeks of gestation and term, even though it shows the same initial decrease as the others that remain depressed.

Pregnant women handle amino acids in an unusual way in their response to starvation. After 84 to 90 hours of starvation (water allowed), valine, leucine, isoleucine, and α-amino butyric acid levels increased twofold to threefold both in 23 pregnant women awaiting termination of pregnancy and in 11 nonpregnant women in a control group. Alanine concentrations decreased in both groups, but the decrease was less in the pregnant subjects. Glycine levels decreased by about 50% in the control subjects, but increased by about 25% in the pregnant women. For those with an interest in obstetric physiology, the study of maternal amino acid changes and their possible significance during pregnancy offers a rich investigative pasture in which to browse.

Uric acid concentrations in serum decrease from a nonpregnancy average value of 3.9 ± 0.74 mg/dl (0.234 ± 0.044 mmol/liter) to 2.9 ± 0.66 mg/dl (0.174 ± 0.039 mmol/liter) at 12 weeks. This reduced level is maintained until about 24 weeks' gestation, but the concentration increases thereafter such that, by term, it is usually above the nonpregnancy value. In the series yielding the values given, the term average was 4.4 ± 0.92 mg/dl (0.264 ± 0.055 mmol/liter). Urine concentrations of uric acid change virtually in parallel, and it seems probable that the changing serum levels of uric acid reflect changes in the amount of uric acid reabsorbed by the proximal renal tubules rather than any change in uric acid metabolism.

The purists argue correctly that the tubular handling of filtered uric acid is complex. Initially, it is absorbed. Further down the proximal tubule, however, some is secreted into the tubular lumen, to be followed by a second reabsorption phase even further down the tubule. The overall effect is that most of the uric acid filtered at the glomerulus is reabsorbed. Small changes in renal handling thus have a marked effect on circulating levels of uric acid. This is of clinical importance because some reports have suggested that increasing levels of circulating uric acid are indicative of preeclampsia; such an interpretation should be made with caution, because these levels normally increase in the third trimester of uncomplicated pregnancies.

VITAMINS

Researchers who wish to investigate the effect of normal pregnancy on vitamin metabolism in the human rather than the animal model face considerable difficulties. Pharmacokinetic studies using vitamins labeled with carbon 14 could provide many answers, but are obviously unsuitable for use in pregnant women. A nonradioactive isotope, such as carbon 13, could be used, but few such vitamin tracers are available; furthermore, the cost of the determinations with mass spectroscopy would be formidable. The more classic depletion–repletion studies are not permissible in pregnant women on either ethical or practical grounds. To obtain a depleted status for vitamin A, for example, might require 300 to 400 days! The only feasible method involves dietary survey and intake studies—which are notoriously inaccurate.

Serum (or urine) levels are totally inadequate for assessing maternal vitamin status, and red cell levels are probably little better as "tissue markers." The following data are therefore generalizations, and clinical diagnoses or management should rarely, if ever, be based on such values alone.

Ascorbic acid concentrations in blood are subject to wide variations, depending on the recent diet. Some broad conclusions can be drawn from a study of a sufficiently large number of women who eat a relatively standard diet, however. One such study of Egyptian women suggested a decrease in the ascorbic acid level from a nonpregnancy value of 9.5 mg/liter to approximately 5.6 mg/liter by term; in American women, there was a decrease from a midpregnancy concentration of 7.5 mg/liter to approximately 3.3 mg/liter by term.

Vitamin B$_6$ concentrations are also lower toward term, and claims have been made that this decrease is due to fetal demand. One study reported a plasma pyridoxal phosphate level of 6.24 μg/liter at the end of the first trimester, decreasing to 1.44 μg/liter by term. When given a tryptophan load, these women excreted an increased amount of xanthurenic acid in their urine. Taken together, these findings suggest a vitamin B_6 deficiency in pregnant subjects. It seems more likely that both findings again reflect the new homeostatic norm for pregnancy.

A single vitamin is usually present in food as a mixture of related substances or "vitamers." In the case of vitamin B_6, for example, these are pyridoxine, pyridoxal, and pyridoxamine, all of which are metabolically processed to the active form in the body. It seems improbable that there is any fetal demand for vitamin B_6 or any other nutrient of such magnitude that it would deplete the supply of an otherwise normal woman and reduce her to deficiency. The fetus does have highly efficient methods for ensuring its own supplies; however, if a woman's diet is nutritionally insufficient, the fetus will rarely be inconvenienced. The fat-soluble vitamins cross the phospholipid membranes of the placental cells by simple diffusion; to ensure this, the maternal blood levels are usually greater than fetal blood levels. The water-soluble vitamins are actively transported across the placenta, and the fetus can therefore deprive the mother, irrespective of her blood levels, which are usually lower than the fetal levels. The generally accepted gradients between the maternal and fetal blood concentrations for the various vitamins are given in Table 1–9; these mothers were not given vitamin supplementation during pregnancy.

CLOTTING FACTORS

A profusion of terms has evolved in regard to the factors governing blood coagulation. One system uses Roman numerals, but unfortunately, the factors are not numbered in the order in which they affect events that result in fibrin formation. The other system is a mixture of the names of investigators and descriptive nouns. The two systems are shown in Table 1–10.

The basic mechanisms of hemostasis are the same in pregnant women as in nonpregnant women, but the concentrations or activity of some of the factors are increased during pregnancy. Thus, when a blood vessel is damaged, Factor XII is activated by collagen (the so-called intrinsic mechanism), while Factor VII is activated by the thromboplastin released by the damaged tissues (the extrinsic

Table 1-9. *Approximate gradients between maternal and fetal blood concentrations for the various vitamins*

Vitamins	Gradients
Vitamin A	1.2:1
Vitamin E	4:1
Ascorbic acid	1:2 (up to 1:3)
Thiamin	1:1.8
Riboflavin	1:2
Nicotinic acid	1:1.5
Folate	1:2.5
Vitamin B_{12}	1:3
Vitamin B_6	1:3 (up to 1:6)

Table 1-10. *Factors involved in blood coagulation and synonyms*

Roman Factor Number	Synonym
I	Fibrinogen
II	Prothrombin
III	Tissue thromboplastin
IV	Calcium ions
V	Proaccelerin
VII	Factor VII
VIII	Antihemophilic factor (AHF)
IX	Christmas factor
X	Stuart or Prower factor
XI	Plasma thromboplastin antecedent (PTA)
XII	Hageman factor
XIII	Fibrin-stabilizing factor

mechanism). Although both the intrinsic and extrinsic pathways are activated by components released from the damaged vessel wall and neither can exist in isolation, this division into two mechanisms is a useful way of describing the rather complicated series of events by which factors present in only picogram amounts activate a sequence of enzyme events that cause milligrams of fibrinogen to become fibrin (Fig. 1–8).

Fibrinogen is the only factor present in amounts sufficiently large to be measured reliably. During pregnancy, concentrations increase from a nonpregnancy average of 250-400 mg/dl to as much as 600 mg/dl by term. The basic molecule consists of three pairs of polypeptide chains linked by disulfide bonds. The proteolytic enzyme thrombin splits off two pairs of smaller peptides, fibrinopeptides A and B, to produce fibrin monomer, which then undergoes polymerization to the insoluble fibrin form. It seems that Factor XIII increases fibrin stability by linking the amino acids in adjacent areas of the separate fibrin fibers.

Factor VII activity may increase as much as tenfold by term; similar increases have been noted in women taking combined oral contraceptive agents.

Factor VIII, the antihemophilic factor, doubles its activity by term. There is some disagreement about Factor VIII and its related antigen; some investigators suggest that both increase to the same proportional extent so that the ratio of the two remains constant, while others have found a greater increase in antigen behavior.

Factors IX and XII both increase their activity during normal pregnancy. The levels of **Factors XI and XIII** decrease, with that of Factor XI falling to as low as 60% of the nonpregnancy value and that of Factor XIII falling to 50% of the nonpregnancy value.

If intravascular changes cause a blood clot to form, the dissemination of the clot beyond the site of tissue injury is prevented by the strict control of thrombin. First, the clot is absorbed onto the fibrin as it is formed (this action is sometimes referred to as antithrombin I); second, the level of **antithrombin III**, a potent

38

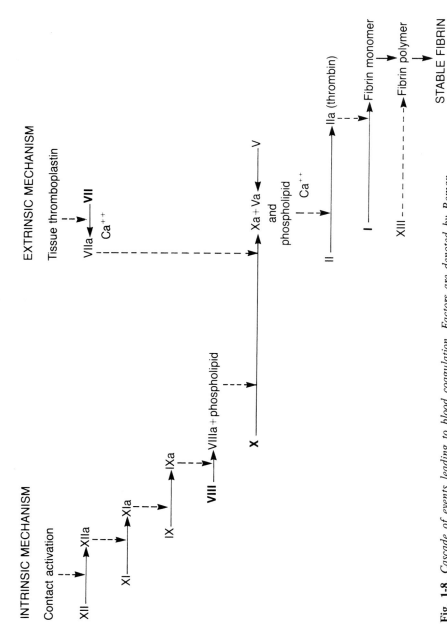

Fig. 1-8. *Cascade of events leading to blood coagulation. Factors are denoted by Roman numerals; those affected by pregnancy are in bold type.*

thrombin inhibitor that is an α_2-globulin contained in the plasma, probably decreases during pregnancy. The gap between these two numbered actions has been filled by a protein known to potentiate the action of heparin; this is sometimes referred to as heparin cofactor, but is more neatly called antithrombin II. An agent said to inhibit activated Factor X (i.e., Xa), not unreasonably called anti-Xa, may be identical to antithrombin III.

These "local" controls that confine the clot to the site of tissue damage are not to be confused with the fibrinolytic system, which has four major components: plasminogen, plasmin, activators, and inhibitors. Plasminogen is a β-globulin that is composed of a single polypeptide chain and is probably synthesized in the liver. It is the inactive precursor of the proteolytic enzyme plasmin. When formed from plasminogen's single polypeptide chain, plasmin becomes a two-chain molecule connected by a disulphide bond. The plasma factors that activate plasmin are highly labile and difficult to measure, since they have a "life" of about 15 minutes. Such naturally occurring activators are found in most human organs, but are concentrated mostly around the blood vessels, especially the veins. Inhibitors are of two main types: antiactivators, which inhibit the transformation of plasminogen to plasmin, and antiplasmins, which inhibit the action of formed plasmin. Platelets have antiplasmin activity, which may be the reason that platelet thrombi can occur.

Normally, the presence of the various inhibitors in the general circulation limit the action of plasmin to the digestion of formed fibrin. However, plasmin can also act on prothrombin, Factors V and VII, glucagon, ACTH, and growth hormone.

Fibrin and fibrinogen degradation products form when these proteins are broken down by plasmin. If we assume a molecular weight of 344,000 for fibrinogen, the first act of plasmin is to split off fragment X, a large fragment with a molecular weight of 240,000, leaving the smaller fragments called A , B and C. Fragment X then divides into fragment Y (molecular weight of 155,000) and D (molecular weight of 83,000). Finally, fragment Y is further divided into more fragment D and E (molecular weight of 50,000). Approximately 70% of fragment X is retained in the clot, however; somewhat less of fragment Y is retained, and only about 10% of fragments D and E are retained. Hence, larger amounts of fragments D and E are found in the circulation relative to fragments X and Y; at the present time, all these fragments appear to be equiantigenic and are recognized by antifibrinogen antibody. The concentration of these degradation products increases progressively throughout pregnancy, but not to levels that would be confused with disseminated intravascular coagulation problems.

It has been suggested that the increase in the fibrinogen concentration during pregnancy must lead to a condition of "hypercoagulability," but both the bleeding time and clotting time are normal in pregnant women. A more physiologic explanation may be that, under normal circulatory conditions, pregnant women do not have any increased tendency to intravascular coagulation, but do have a much improved capacity to respond to initiating events, such as separation of the placenta during the third stage of labor. The fact that venous stasis, which tends to occur in the legs by the third trimester of pregnancy, is another initiating event may explain the increased incidence of deep venous thrombosis in pregnant women. It is also probable that plasma fibrinolytic activity is decreased during pregnancy and labor, but it appears to return to nonpregnancy levels within an hour of the placenta delivery. This suggests that the placenta mediates this inhibition, probably by producing fibrinolytic inhibitors.

2
Cardiovascular System

Heart

Size: Increases by about 12%.

Murmurs: Both systolic and diastolic occur and are physiologic.

ECG: Changes similar in some respects to cardiac ischemia, but are *due to positional changes* in the heart.

Rhythm: Extrasystoles common and *supraventricular tachycardia* not unusual.

Cardiac output: Increases by approximately 1.5 liter/min to term.

Heart rate: Increases from about 70 to 85 beats/min.

Stroke volume: Increases from about 63 to 70 ml.

Arteriovenous oxygen difference: Decreases by the end of the first trimester from approximately 44 ml/liter to 33 ml/liter, but *increases* toward term to nonpregnancy levels.

Blood Pressure

Arterial blood pressure: Systolic probably unchanged by pregnancy, but *diastolic decreases* during midpregnancy and gradually *increases* after 26 to 28 weeks to nonpregnancy values by term.

Pulse pressure: Is higher than average during midpregnancy.

Venous pressure: Remains *unchanged* in the arms, but significantly *increased* in the femoral venous system.

Peripheral resistance (mean arterial blood pressure divided by cardiac output): Decreases.

Pulmonary blood pressure: Unchanged from nonpregnancy values.

Circulation time: Appears to be *unchanged.*

Blood Flow Distribution

Uterus: Increased, possibly by 500 ml/min.

Kidneys: Increased by approximately 400 ml/min.

Skin: Increased by perhaps 300 to 400 ml/min.

Liver: Probably *unchanged,* but definitive human data awaited.

Breasts: Increased perhaps by 200 ml or so.

Cerebral flow: Unchanged from nonpregnancy values.

Gut and spleen: Probably *increased* slightly, but data awaited.

Techniques for measuring different aspects of cardiovascular dynamics are necessarily indirect, complex, and extremely difficult to standardize. Apparent conflicts in previous reports concerned with cardiovascular changes associated with pregnancy are usually the result of differences in the measurement conditions and techniques rather than true pregnancy adaptations. Some of these difficulties are unresolved today.

HEART

The **size** of the heart appears to increase by about 12%, according to radiologic measurements. This would increase the capacity of the heart by 70 to 80 ml if the total increase was accorded to diastolic filling, but there is also some degree of cardiac muscle hypertrophy.

Murmurs are usually physiologic, but they must be listened to with some care so that minor degrees of cardiac disease are not overlooked. Systolic murmurs, commonly called ejection murmurs, are attributed to the increased stroke volume; they usually occur in early or middle systole and are best heard along the left sternal edge. Occasionally, apparent systolic murmurs are heard over the base of the heart, but these originate from the mammary arteries.

A diastolic murmur can be detected in some women. Again best heard along the left sternal edge, this murmur is sometimes coincident with the third heart sound. It is often transient in nature, which helps to distinguish it from those originating from a true valvular pathology.

The **ECG** changes, mainly because of the positional shift in the heart. The gradual elevation of the diaphragm causes the heart to be pushed upward and forward, the apex beat coming to lie in the fourth rather than the fifth intercostal space; the electrical axis deviates to the left by 15° to 20°. In general, there are no Q waves in lead aV_F; in many women, the T wave is flattened or even inverted in lead III. Such changes should not be confused with cardiac ischemia.

Heart **rhythm** is often irregular, since atrial and ventricular extrasystoles are common and supraventricular tachycardia is not infrequent.

Cardiac output determinations have been hindered by methodologic differences and a failure by earlier investigators to appreciate that women lying on their back during late pregnancy are likely to have a reduced venous return to the heart. It can now be stated with reasonable confidence, however, that cardiac output increases to its maximum within the first trimester and that this increase is maintained to term. Output increases by about 1.5 liter/min above the nonpregnancy average, and it seems unlikely that this value decreases between 32 weeks and term as earlier work suggested.

Heart rate increases by about 15 beats/min if the sleeping pulse rate is used (i.e., from about 70 to 85 beats/min). Of all the measurements, rate is the most prone to be affected by such factors as anxiety, emotional stress, exercise, and heat; even the sleeping pulse may be affected if the act of recording it disturbs the patient. These data were obtained as the averages of continuous overnight monitoring, however.

According to traditional teaching, **stroke volume** also increases. Data are usually derived from simultaneous measurements of cardiac output and rate, and the conditions of measurement and the rapid changes that occur in rate may alter the day-to-day average stroke volume. Indeed, women with artificial pacemakers that give them a fixed normal heart rate appear to undergo pregnancy without problems. If output increases from approximately 4.5 to 6 liter/min and rate increases from 70 to 85 beats/min, however, this must be achieved by an increase in stroke volume from about 63 to 70 ml.

The **arteriovenous oxygen difference**, expressed as the difference between the level of oxygen in arterial blood as it leaves the heart and that in venous blood as it returns to the heart, should decrease if these data are correct. Although, as noted earlier, cardiac output is maximal within the first trimester, maternal and fetal oxygen requirements are not greatly increased at this stage; venous blood therefore is more oxygenated, and the arteriovenous oxygen difference is smaller. The average nonpregnancy value is 44 ml/liter, but the value decreases to approximately 33 ml/liter during the first trimester and gradually increases toward the nonpregnancy value or perhaps just exceeds it by term.

BLOOD PRESSURE

It is almost impossible to compare **arterial blood pressure** data from different centers because such factors as the width of the inflatable cuff used, the speed with which the manometer mercury column is allowed to fall, the position and state of rest of the patient, the thickness of her arm, and interobserver recording error have marked effects on blood pressure readings. Despite these difficulties and the consequent unavailability of meaningful values for systolic and diastolic blood pressures during normal pregnancy, there is broad agreement on their patterns of change: relatively little change in systolic blood pressure throughout pregnancy, but a reduction in diastolic blood pressure from about 12 to 26 weeks, increasing thereafter to reach the nonpregnancy value by 36 weeks or so. As a result, **pulse pressure** is higher than average during midpregnancy.

Posture has a profound effect. If a pregnant woman lies on her back during late pregnancy, the weight of her uterus not only may compress her inferior vena cava, causing profound supine hypotension, but also may partially compress her aorta, causing the femoral arterial blood pressure to fall below the brachial arterial pressure. Similarly, the arm blood pressure recorded while a pregnant woman is lying down (supine) may appear to rise if she is asked to roll onto one side and her blood pressure is re-recorded. This is due in part to the fact that the recording cuff position is now physically elevated some 10 cm above the plane of the heart (equivalent to about 7 mm Hg).

For all practical purposes, there are no valves between the femoral veins and the heart; if a nonpregnant woman lies down, the pressure in these veins is similar to that in the right atrium. During pregnancy, however, there is a marked increase in femoral **venous pressure**, while atrial pressure remains unchanged. The implication is that an obstruction must be present between these veins and the heart when pregnant patients lie down. The weight of the pregnant uterus on the inferior vena cava, the pressure of the fetal head on the common iliac veins, and a high pressure venous return from the uterine veins causing a hemodynamic "back pressure" below their inflow are all possible causes. Venous pressure does not change in the arm veins.

Peripheral resistance is defined as mean arterial blood pressure divided by cardiac output. As the former is little affected by pregnancy, but cardiac output increases, then resistance must fall. It has been calculated that the nonpregnancy value of 1,300 dynes/sec/cm^{-5} decreases to approximately 979 dynes/sec/cm^{-5} by midpregnancy.

Pulmonary blood pressure might be expected to increase during early pregnancy, as the pulmonary artery is one of the recipients of the increased cardiac output; however, the pressure in the right ventricle, the pulmonary artery, and its capillaries is unchanged. This suggests that pulmonary resistance to flow decreases by dilatation of its vascular bed. In addition, there is radiologic evidence indicating increased lung vascularity.

Circulation time appears unchanged during pregnancy, although the methods used to determine circulation time are relatively imprecise (e.g., the time required for a bolus of dye to travel from an antecubital vein to a photoelectric cell detector placed over the lobe of the ear).

BLOOD FLOW DISTRIBUTION

That the blood flow to various organs, such as the uterus and breasts, should increase during pregnancy seems logical. The mechanisms that control such changes are little understood, however; certainly, they must be complex. For example, when a vascular bed increases in volume, cardiac output must also increase if blood pressure is to be maintained.

Blood flow to the **uterus** undoubtedly increases, but the precise amount depends on the stage of gestation at which it is determined. By term, an estimate of 500 ml/min is probably reasonable, but values as high as 700 to 800 ml/min have been reported.

Measurements of renal blood flow are rather more precise and therefore more reliable. Blood flow to the **kidneys** increases to approximately 400 ml/min above the nonpregnancy average. Some investigators have postulated that renal blood flow decreases toward term, but this is unlikely; measurements that suggested such a decrease were usually made with the patient supine, which probably caused an artifactual decrease during the third trimester because of caval compression.

The **skin** has an increased blood flow during pregnancy, particularly over the hands and feet. One possible reason for this is to allow the mother to radiate away the excess body heat that results from her increased metabolism. Skin blood flow patterns cannot be generalized, however; the increase to the skin of the forearm and calf, if any, is certainly less than that to the hands and feet; smoking affects blood flow to the skin, as does ambient temperature at the time the determinations are made. Again, generalizations must be made, and an overall figure of 300 to 400 ml/min is probably reasonable.

Some investigators have suggested that **liver** blood flow is unchanged at 1,400 to 1,500 ml/min, corrected for a body surface area of 1.73 m^2. Others have reported an increase from the nonpregnancy average of 800 ml/min to a pregnancy maximum of about 1,400 ml/min. Because of the liver's vital role in general metabolism and the considerable metabolic adjustments demanded by pregnancy, it seems reasonable that the blood flow would increase; reliable human data are still awaited, however. For the moment, it must be assumed that flow to the liver does not increase.

The breasts have an increased blood supply, but because they are enlarged during pregnancy, precise determinations are difficult. Many pregnant women are aware of dilated veins coursing over the surface of their breasts, however, and a figure of about 200 ml/min may be a realistic estimate.

It has been suggested that the blood flow to other sites, such as to the **spleen** and the **gut**, is also increased, but data are lacking; **cerebral blood flow** is not increased above nonpregnancy values.

In summary, it has been suggested that uterine blood flow accounts for approximately 500 ml/min; renal blood flow, approximately 400 ml/min; the skin, approximately 300 ml/min; and the breasts, approximately 200 ml/min. If other sites account for about 100 ml/min (or if liver blood flow is increased), these generalized values account for the 1.5 liter/min increase in cardiac output.

3

Renal System

Renal Anatomy

Body surface area: It is *inappropriate to correct* serial renal data throughout pregnancy to the usual 1.73 m^2.

Anatomic changes: Renal length appears to *increase* by about 1 cm. Renal calyces and ureters *dilate* and may contain 40 to 100 ml in total.

Renal Dynamics

Effective renal plasma flow: Increases by 50% or more from a nonpregnancy average of about 480 ml/min to 890 ml/min or more.

Glomerular filtration rate (GFR): Increases from a nonpregnancy average of 97 ml/min to 128 ml/min by 10 weeks of gestation; there may be a small *decrease* between 36 weeks of gestation and term.

Homeostatic Control

Acid–base balance: pH increases from 7.40 to 7.44.

Potassium: About *350 mEq is retained* in the course of pregnancy.

Sodium: About *950 mEq is accumulated* throughout pregnancy.

Urinary output: 24-hour volume is largely *unchanged.*

Posture: Changes in posture cause only short-term effect on the kidneys' ability to handle water and sodium.

Excretion of Nutrients

Glucose: Excreted in increasing amounts, but the pattern of glycosuria and amount excreted per 24 hours appear to be random.

Other sugars: All excreted in *increased* amounts, except arabinose.

Amino acids: Total amount excreted is *increased,* but variation among the individual amino acids.

Vitamins: Water-soluble forms are *excreted in greater amounts.*

Protein: 24-hour total excretion usually *unchanged.*

Renin–Angiotensin System

Renin: Circulating levels are *increased.*

Substrate: The α_2-macroglobulin is *increased* in blood.

Angiotensins I and II: Both present in the circulation in *increased* amounts.

Vascular response: Is *diminished* so that the pressor effect anticipated from the increase in AII does not occur.

The kidneys are involved in many pregnancy disorders, but the researcher interested in human pregnancy and its complications faces many obstacles in studying renal function. There is no useful animal model against which to compare humans with respect to renal function during pregnancy; in the dog and rat, animals used to describe so many renal changes, glomerular filtration rate (GFR) increases by only 10% to 15%, and effective renal plasma flow probably does not increase at all.

The term *glomerular filtration rate* refers to the volume of plasma completely cleared of a particular solute per minute. The ideal solute not only would be completely filtered at the glomerulus, but also would not be secreted, absorbed, or metabolized by the renal tubules. It would be stable in urine so that it could be assayed some time after collection, and the methods for its assay would be both sensitive and specific. These characteristics are only half the problem, however; the other half is the patient. Ideally, she must be able to empty her bladder and her ureters completely each time she micturates so that filtered solute retained in the dead space of the collecting system and hence not assayed in the timed urine sample volume will not cause calculation errors. This "loss" can be kept to an effective minimum by maintaining a high urine flow rate over the time of the collection, which reduces the volume of the dead space, proportionally, to a small part of the total urine volume. While the patients can be encouraged to drink with this aim in mind, IV fluid loading must be avoided because expansion of the vascular volume itself affects GFR.

The carbohydrate inulin has many of the characteristics of the ideal solute for filtration studies. It is freely filtered, but not reabsorbed, secreted, nor metabolized by the tubules. Unfortunately, it must be given by IV infusion, and it tends to precipitate from urine if allowed to cool. Endogenous creatinine clearance is more commonly used, but the clearance period should be at least 12, and preferably 24, hours. Furthermore, the patients must be meticulous in ensuring that they obtain a complete collection. A single blood sample is usually considered sufficiently representative of the blood concentration over the entire 24-hour period, but this is an assumption. Because of these potential difficulties in undertaking even a relatively "simple" renal function test, reliable data concerned with renal changes induced by pregnancy are relatively sparse.

RENAL ANATOMY

Body Surface Area

The size of the kidneys is thought to be related to body size. In order to compare the renal function of individuals as widely varied in size as children and adults, it has become conventional to express renal clearance data in terms of body surface area. Since 1928, the accepted figure for the body surface area of a 25-year-old man has been 1.73 m^2, and this has been the value to which all data obtained since that date have been referred. It is illogical to make such a correction for serial data on a single patient throughout pregnancy since the woman's height is constant and the major part of her weight gain is the product of conception rather than change in maternal body mass.

Anatomic Changes

The kidneys appear to increase by approximately 1 cm in length during pregnancy, but renal biopsy studies have suggested that the microscopic structure of the renal tissue is unchanged. Renal weight is also increased, according to the relatively sparse necropsy data available. The overall conclusion seems to be that the renal changes indicate an increased water content.

The renal calyces are dilated, as are the ureters down to the level of the pelvic brim. These changes can significantly increase the renal dead space; the right ureter can contain 20 to 50 ml urine, and the left ureter perhaps slightly less. Contrary to popular belief, the muscular tone of the ureters is not reduced and may indeed be slightly increased during pregnancy. Obstruction at the level of the pelvic brim is not likely to be caused by pressure from the iliac arteries, increased venous tone in the vessels around the ureters, or the weight of the uterus, because signs of obstruction are rarely seen in association with nonpregnancy causes of uterine enlargement, such as fibroids. Probably all of the postulated endocrinologic and anatomic causes contribute to pregnancy changes in the urinary tract. Radiologic evidence suggests that these pregnancy changes do not completely resolve until 12 to 16 weeks postdelivery.

RENAL DYNAMICS

Effective Renal Plasma Flow

The changes in the effective renal plasma flow have a history not dissimilar to that of cardiac output. Early cross-sectional data suggested a gradual increase

Table 3-1. *Effective renal plasma flow (ml/min) determined by* p-*aminohippurate (PAH) clearance in 25 healthy women*

	Nonpregnant (8–10 Weeks Postpartum)	Gestation (weeks)		
		16	*26*	*36*
Mean	479.8	840.5	891.2	770.8
± SD	72.0	144.7	278.9	175.4

in effective renal plasma flow that reached a maximum at 12 to 16 weeks of gestation and decreased between 36 weeks of gestation and term. Recent serial data obtained with *p*-aminohippurate (PAH) suggest that maximum flow is achieved by the end of the second trimester and is maintained until term with little, if any, effect brought about by a change in posture. Absolute values depend on the methods used for their determination; in percentage terms, however, increases of 50% to 80% above nonpregnancy values can be anticipated in women who offer their own nonpregnancy control data. In one serial study of 25 healthy women, their nonpregnancy (8 weeks postpartum) mean value was 479 ± 72 ml/min, increasing to a maximum value of 891 ± 279 ml/min at 26 weeks of gestation (Table 3–1). There is still some controversy concerning whether the effective renal plasma flow decreases toward term or whether the data that suggest such a decrease indicate postural effects. If there is a genuine decrease, it is probably small.

Glomerular Filtration Rate

It appears that the GFR has a biphasic change during normal pregnancy when determined as 24-hour endogenous creatinine clearance. In 36 women studied serially from prior to conception to term, the average prepregnancy GFR was 97 ml/min, increasing to 125 ml/min by 20 weeks and remaining at this level to 36 weeks. At 38 weeks, the average decreased somewhat (Table 3–2). While this change was relatively small, it appeared to be consistent within patients, suggesting a complex series of events in renal dynamics throughout pregnancy.

The mother is not responding to fetal demand, because maximal maternal renal adaptations occur within the first third of pregnancy when fetal metabolic

Table 3-2. *GFR (ml/min) determined from endogenous creatinine clearance in healthy women studied serially throughout pregnancy*

	Prepregnancy	Gestation (weeks)							
		6	*10*	*16*	*20*	*28*	*32*	*36*	*38*
Mean	97.18	112.7	126.0	122.2	125.2	128.5	134.7	133.7	128.1
± SD	16.1	14.3	20.8	18.5	27.0	24.4	22.4	24.2	24.9
Number	36	31	31	36	36	36	34	36	36

needs must be small. Furthermore, when fetal size is greatest, the GFR does not increase and may even decrease somewhat toward term. As the values in Table 3–2 were determined over 24 hours, it seems unlikely that such a decrease reflects any effect of posture or normal exercise. Although a small but variable quantity of creatinine is secreted by the renal tubules so that the total appearing in the urine is somewhat more than the amount filtered, the degree of increase in the GFR is much greater than can be accounted for by the increased urinary creatinine content from tubular secretion alone.

The mechanism by which the GFR increases is not understood, but it may be simply a reflection of the increase in the effective renal plasma flow. This is no explanation, however, because it is not known what governs the change in the effective renal plasma flow. It is tempting to speculate that, because the plasma albumin concentration decreases during the first trimester and the GFR increases maximally over the same period, one causes the other. The reduced level of albumin in the plasma reaching the glomerular capillary would reduce the oncotic pressure, and it would thus take longer to offset the hydraulic pressure in the vessel (i.e., the GFR would increase). Blood pressure also decreases during pregnancy, however. While no data are available concerning the efferent arteriolar tone in the human glomerulus, it seems simplistic to expect the explanation to be in such a simple balance.

The spectrum of endocrinologic changes in pregnancy has been invoked as a cause of the increased GFR, and various hormones may in fact play a part. Progesterone has been cited in particular; but in one study in which it was given to nonpregnant patients in doses meant to induce pregnancy concentrations, it had little effect on the GFR—although the effective renal plasma flow did increase initially.

HOMEOSTATIC CONTROL

The human internal environment is largely maintained by the efficiency of the kidneys in regulating the volumes of various fluid compartments and their biochemical composition.

Acid–Base Balance

During pregnancy, the mean arterial P_{CO_2} decreases from approximately 39 mm Hg to approximately 30 to 31 mm Hg. The blood levels of hydrogen ion also decrease somewhat (2 to 4 mEq/liter), and plasma bicarbonate concentrations decrease by some 4 mEq/liter so that values in the range 18 to 22 mEq/liter are the pregnancy norm. The effect of these changes is that arterial pH averages 7.44 in pregnant patients compared with 7.40 in nonpregnant patients.

Potassium

Pregnant women appear to have an enhanced ability to retain potassium. It might be expected that their more alkaline urine, together with the marked increase in their blood levels of aldosterone and other mineralocorticoids, would lead to an enhanced excretion of potassium, but such is not the case. Indeed, an additional 350 mEq or so of potassium is retained throughout pregnancy; this resistance of pregnant women to kaliuresis has been ascribed to the action of progesterone.

Sodium

Total body water increases by about 8 liters during pregnancy, the majority being held in the extracellular compartment. As its biochemical composition is essentially the same as that of the nonpregnant woman and sodium is the major solute, a considerable amount of sodium must be retained; about 950 mEq is accumulated throughout pregnancy. Renal reabsorption of sodium is increased, and the energy required for this increased tubular work accounts for a major proportion of the metabolic cost of pregnancy. If an average nonpregnancy serum sodium concentration is 139 mEq/liter and the GFR is 100 ml/min, then 20,016 mEq sodium is filtered each day; of these, about 140 mEq is excreted (i.e., a reabsorption efficiency of 99.3%). During pregnancy, if the GFR is 150 ml/min and the serum sodium value is decreased to 136 mEq/liter, then 29,376 mEq sodium is filtered each day, yet only about 166 mEq is lost in the urine per day (Table 3–3). Thus, despite an increase of about 47% in the amount of sodium presented to the renal tubules every 24 hours, their reabsorption efficiency is maintained at better than 99%. These adaptations are completed by the end of the first trimester.

Urinary Output

Interestingly, this marked increase in the GFR is not reflected in the 24-hour urinary output, which changes little, if any, throughout pregnancy. Data obtained from 36 healthy women who collected 24-hour urine samples regularly throughout pregnancy showed no significant increase in the volume of urine passed per day as pregnancy progressed (Table 3–4). Thus, the increased filtered load of water is reabsorbed with equal efficiency when required.

Posture

Much has been made of the effect of posture on the ability of the kidneys to handle water and sodium. Traditional teaching suggests that, when a pregnant

Table 3-3. *Fasting plasma sodium concentrations and 24-hour urinary sodium excretion values in 9 healthy women studied during a preconception menstrual cycle then serially to 16 weeks of gestation*

	Plasma Sodium (mEq/liter)	24-Hour Sodium Excretion (mEq)
Menstrual cycle		
Week 1	140.4 ± 1.4	136 ± 38
2	139.0 ± 1.2	126 ± 33
3	138.7 ± 0.7	166 ± 42
4	140.4 ± 1.7	148 ± 38
Pregnancy		
Week 2	138.9 ± 2.1	121 ± 31
3	138.6 ± 2.4	166 ± 41
4	139.6 ± 1.1	158 ± 40
5	139.1 ± 1.7	171 ± 45
6	138.6 ± 1.3	176 ± 48
7	137.6 ± 2.5	174 ± 40
8	137.1 ± 2.1	178 ± 50
9	137.7 ± 2.6	174 ± 49
10	136.2 ± 3.4	169 ± 46
11	136.2 ± 3.2	173 ± 44
12	136.3 ± 1.9	175 ± 60
13	136.1 ± 1.7	170 ± 53
14	135.8 ± 3.2	158 ± 51
15	136.4 ± 2.7	160 ± 54
16	136.6 ± 1.5	162 ± 51

Table 3-4. *24-Hour urinary volumes in 36 healthy women studied at regular intervals throughout pregnancy*

Gestation (weeks)	Number	24-Hour Urinary Volume (ml)
1	11	1516 ± 554
2	11	1516 ± 398
3	23	1380 ± 469
4	26	1425 ± 376
6	26	1351 ± 386
8	29	1434 ± 421
10	36	1399 ± 425
12	36	1505 ± 428
16	36	1421 ± 446
20	36	1532 ± 551
24	36	1456 ± 418
28	36	1596 ± 373
32	36	1588 ± 489
36	36	1580 ± 503
38	33	1511 ± 454

woman changes from a lateral recumbent position to the supine position or stands upright, there is a reduction in urine flow, GFR, and effective renal plasma flow. In particular, it has been argued that any change of posture during renal function studies undertaken during the last trimester alters the urine flow and hence leads to inaccurate results. Now, however, it seems probable that changes in posture do not cause other than very short-term effects. From a physiologic viewpoint, a healthy pregnant woman is mobile and hence changes her posture frequently during a day. Keeping patients at rest during renal function studies is likely to lead to results that are accurately determined in scientific terms, but are physiologically false.

Posture is bound to have an overall influence; because of gravitational and hydrostatic forces, together with the decreased osmotic effect from plasma protein concentration, it could be anticipated that water and its isotonic solute content would be "lost" to the extravascular compartment, particularly in the lower limbs. This relative hypovolemia is corrected when the pregnant woman lies down in bed at night and returns this isotonic solution to the intravascular space. This might account, in part, for the troublesome nocturia experienced by some pregnant women.

EXCRETION OF NUTRIENTS

Virtually nothing that is filtered at the glomerulus is reabsorbed by the tubules with 100% efficiency, but the detection of a given substance in urine depends on the sensitivity and specificity of the laboratory methods available. As such methods improve, compounds not previously thought to be present in urine are being "found."

Glucose

It was once believed that glucose was not present in the urine of healthy people, and its detection inevitably made the physician ponder the possibility of diabetes mellitus. Since the advent of paper reagent strips on which the specific enzyme glucose oxidase produces a color reaction in the presence of glucose, it has become accepted that glycosuria is commonplace. The highly specific hexokinase technique indicates that glycosuria occurs in everyone.

The average male and nonpregnant female excretes 100 to 200 mg (0.55 to 1.1 mmol) glucose per 24 hours. If the GFR is 100 ml/min and the blood glucose over the same period averages 100 mg/dl, some 144 g glucose are filtered over 24 hours, of which 200 mg may be excreted. This, a 99.9% reabsorption efficiency, is even better than sodium reabsorption efficiency, but a detectable amount of glucose remains in the urine. If the average GFR in pregnancy is 150 ml/min, but the average blood glucose value for the 24 hours decreases to 80 mg/dl, the total filtered load of glucose still increases—to about 173 g/24 hours—and hence more glucose appears in the urine. In fact, the amount of glucose excreted each day during pregnancy varies widely, not only between individuals, but also within individuals from occasion to occasion, leading to the large standard deviations shown in Table 3–5.

In order to investigate the pattern of glycosuria more thoroughly, women were given freshly manufactured reagent strips for detecting glucose in urine at a concentration of 40 mg/100 ml or more and asked to test each sample of urine they passed for the 7 consecutive days preceding each antenatal visit. These patients averaged 12 visits each, so there were 12 complete weeks of sampling at regular intervals throughout pregnancy. No consistent pattern emerged; the amount of glucose excreted throughout any day was not related to the time of day, time of eating meals, day of the week, or stage of pregnancy.

It is impossible to describe any typical pattern for glucose excretion during normal pregnancy; however, it appears that approximately 50% of women excrete 500 mg/24 hours or more at some time during pregnancy, and many excrete 1 to 5 g/24 hours without any evidence of disordered carbohydrate metabolism. The reason that glucose is excreted in these varying amounts in an apparently random pattern and presumably unrelated to the plasma glucose levels (i.e., unrelated to meal times) is unclear, but it is clear that testing for glycosuria to screen an antenatal population for diabetes mellitus is not appropriate.

Other Sugars

Arabinose does not appear to be excreted in increased amounts during pregnancy, but the urinary concentrations of lactose, fructose, ribose, xylose, and fucose are elevated. In the past, excess lactose (presumably from the mammary gland) sometimes interfered with nonspecific tests for urinary "sugar," but the advent of reagent strips with specific enzymes, such as glucose oxidase, has eliminated this problem.

Amino Acids

It is possible to generalize and say that the urine of pregnant women contains more amino acids than does that of nonpregnant women, but the exact amounts and excretion patterns of the individual amino acids are difficult to specify. There is considerable variation not only between individuals, but also within individuals from occasion to occasion.

One serial study of ten healthy women having uncomplicated pregnancies revealed three broad patterns of excretion. The excretion rate of one group of amino acids, composed of glycine, histidine, threonine, serine, and alanine, doubled by 16 weeks of pregnancy, increasing thereafter to values approximately fivefold greater than the nonpregnancy average by term. A second group, composed of lysine,

Table 3-5. *Glucose excreted per 24 hours in 36 healthy women studied serially throughout pregnancy*

Gestation (weeks)	Number of Patients	Glucose Excreted per 24 Hours	
		(mmol)	*(mg)*
1	11	0.29 ± 0.05	52 ± 9
2	11	0.29 ± 0.05	52 ± 9
3	23	0.30 ± 0.07	54 ± 13
4	26	0.34 ± 0.09	61 ± 16
6	26	0.54 ± 0.61	97 ± 110
8	29	2.07 ± 7.04	373 ± 1267
10	36	2.04 ± 6.81	367 ± 1226
12	36	3.72 ± 15.40	670 ± 2772
16	36	1.70 ± 4.35	306 ± 783
20	36	3.61 ± 12.10	650 ± 2178
24	36	2.66 ± 7.10	479 ± 1278
28	36	4.48 ± 13.64	806 ± 2455
32	36	5.88 ± 15.80	1058 ± 2844
36	36	4.63 ± 14.56	833 ± 2621
38	33	5.43 ± 21.07	977 ± 3793

cystine, taurine, phenylalanine, valine, leucine, and tyrosine also displayed a rapid increase in excretion during the first 16 weeks or so, but decreased slightly thereafter to term. The amino acids of the third group displayed minimal changes in excretion; glutamic acid, methionine, and ornithine showed a marginal increase during pregnancy relative to their nonpregnancy averages, while asparagine, isoleucine, and arginine showed no change or a marginal decrease (Table 3–6). These patterns are difficult to ascribe to any reasonable physiologic mechanism, and the explanation remains obscure at the present time.

Vitamins

Even allowing for the known increase in GFR, there is a proportionally greater excretion of folate, B_{12}, and ascorbic acid during pregnancy. The reason that these valuable nutrients should be "lost" to the mother remains an enigma. While it can be argued reasonably that the losses are unlikely to affect a well-nourished mother living in a developed country, these losses, particularly the loss of amino acids, could be a source of further nutritional depletion in mothers in underprivileged societies.

Protein

Urinary protein loss changes little, if at all, during normal pregnancy; it averages 200 to 300 mg/24 hours. Increases up to approximately 500 mg/24 hours

Table 3-6. *Urinary excretion of amino acids (μmol/24 hour) in 10 healthy women having uncomplicated pregnancies*

Amino Acids	Up to 20 Weeks	20–29 Weeks	30 Weeks and Over	8 Weeks Postpartum
Alanine	785 ± 208	1227 ± 559	1383 ± 355	265 ± 82
Arginine	21 ± 22	18 ± 17	20 ± 12	27 ± 19
Asparagine	73 ± 47	58 ± 30	91 ± 68	88 ± 140
Cystine	222 ± 422	256 ± 349	111 ± 50	106 ± 59
Glutamic acid	53 ± 19	64 ± 19	66 ± 30	43 ± 22
Glycine	3507 ± 1409	4723 ± 1576	4888 ± 1336	1314 ± 700
Histidine	2874 ± 778	3832 ± 1283	3583 ± 935	685 ± 421
Isoleucine	37 ± 27	43 ± 24	46 ± 19	42 ± 21
Leucine	92 ± 45	77 ± 47	71 ± 38	22 ± 20
Lysine	588 ± 455	501 ± 499	294 ± 187	267 ± 165
Methionine	63 ± 60	83 ± 39	71 ± 32	34 ± 25
Ornithine	122 ± 95	172 ± 187	176 ± 175	116 ± 115
Phenylalanine	114 ± 59	113 ± 80	99 ± 53	48 ± 29
Serine	940 ± 361	1460 ± 887	1523 ± 720	381 ± 166
Taurine	253 ± 167	182 ± 201	98 ± 41	61 ± 35
Threonine	1536 ± 452	2691 ± 1585	2656 ± 1092	442 ± 194
Tyrosine	248 ± 145	256 ± 165	227 ± 102	74 ± 42
Valine	115 ± 145	94 ± 56	99 ± 50	38 ± 20
Totals	11643	15850	15502	4053

may be associated with urinary tract infections and usually involve albumin, transferrin, and γ-globulin. With hypertensive complications of pregnancy, during which protein losses may be recorded as g/24 hours, transferrin, hemopexin, α_1-globulin, α_2-globulin, and γ-globulin may appear in the urine. More severe disorders can be associated with the appearance of α_2-macroglobulins and various immunoglobulin fractions.

RENIN–ANGIOTENSIN SYSTEM

The highly specific enzyme renin found in the circulation has an unusual status during pregnancy. In the nonpregnant woman, renin acts on its substrate angiotensinogen, formed in the liver, to produce first angiotensin I (AI), then angiotensin II (AII), a powerful vasoconstricting agent.

During normal pregnancy, the level of circulating renin begins to increase during the early first trimester and continues to increase progressively until term, achieving values five to ten times greater than nonpregnancy concentrations in some individuals. Like most globulin fractions, angiotensinogen also increases; it rises from a mean nonpregnancy value of 0.7 mg/liter to a mean peak of 3.26 mg/liter. As might be anticipated, the concentrations of AI and AII also increase, but the anticipated effects, vasoconstriction and consequent rise in blood pressure, do not occur. Indeed, pregnant women are remarkably resistant to the pressor effect of infused angiotensin from as early as 10 weeks' gestation.

Several explanations have been advanced for a pregnant woman's lack of responsiveness to angiotensin. The increased production of prostaglandins, which are vasodilatory, or an elevation in the levels of the specific enzyme angiotensinase have been offered as explanations, for example. Whatever the reason, the usual renin–angiotensin balance is maintained over a new fulcrum. Normally, AII levels exert a self-controlling feedback effect by inhibiting renin production, but levels of renin remain elevated in pregnancy despite the increase in AII. Interestingly, the physiologic stimuli that normally produce a renin response in nonpregnant women also produce such a response in pregnant women; sodium restriction and changes in posture stimulate further renin release above the already elevated levels in pregnant women. The decrease in vascular response seems to be specific to AII, as the responses to exogenous norepinephrine are unaltered.

An enzyme that is apparently similar to renin is found in the human uterus, and very high concentrations are present in amniotic fluid. It appears to originate in the cells of the myometrium and chorion, but whether it is identical to circulating renal renin or an isoenzyme is not yet clear. It has also been suggested that some of the circulating (and amniotic fluid) renin is in an inactive form and a high-molecular-weight (or "big renin") form. There is much that remains to be clarified about these enzyme–substrate relations during pregnancy.

4

Endocrine System

Pituitary Gland

Anatomy: Becomes 50% heavier than average adult male.

Prolactin: Increases from about 300 mIU/liter to 5,000 mIU/liter or more by term.

FSH and LH: Suppressed to *low or undetectable* levels during pregnancy.

hGH: Reduced and not responsive to usual stimuli (e.g., insulin-induced hypoglycemia).

Somatomedin C: May be *increased* slightly or remain unchanged.

ACTH: Modestly *increased* during pregnancy, despite the increased cortisol levels.

TSH: Unchanged during pregnancy and apparently responsive to injected thyrotropin-releasing hormone.

MSH: Increased perhaps 100-fold during normal gestation.

Arginine vasopressin: Probably *unchanged* in concentration and responsiveness.

Oxytocin: Unchanged and probably *unaffected by labor.*

Thyroid Gland

Anatomy: Does not change.

TBG: Doubles by the end of the first trimester, nearly *triples* by term.

Thyroxine (T_4): The amount of total circulating T_4 *increases.* The free fraction is probably *unchanged,* but may increase slightly.

Triiodothyronine (T_3): Total amount *increases,* but the free fraction is probably *unchanged.*

Reverse T_3: The amount is *unchanged* in maternal circulation, but *increased* in cord blood.

Adrenal Hormones

Anatomy: Does not change.

CBG: More than doubles by the second trimester.

Cortisol: Increased some threefold above nonpregnancy values, and its episodic pattern of release is probably maintained.

Aldosterone: Increased twofold or more by term.

Deoxycorticosterone (DOC): Increased about 20-fold and as much as 100-fold by term in some women.

Testosterone: The total amount *increased,* but the free fraction appears to be *reduced.*

Androstenedione: Increased by about 50% at term, and its rate of transformation to estradiol and estrone increased about tenfold.

Dehydroepiandrosterone (DHEA): Either *unaltered* or perhaps undergoing a small *decrease* during pregnancy.

Catecholamines: Epinephrine, norepinephrine and dopamine appear to be *unchanged* in normal, unstressed pregnant women, although there may be a small *decrease* in circulating levels of epinephrine.

Islet Cells of the Pancreas

Anatomy: Hypertrophy of the islets, largely resulting from *hyperplasia* of the B cells.

Insulin: Fasting values *increased* by term. Rate of disappearance from the circulation is *unaltered.*

Glucagon: Fasting values *increased,* but proportionally less than insulin so that on an equimolar basis the ratio of insulin to glucagon *increases* during pregnancy.

Somatostatin: Effects *unknown.*

Calcium Regulation

Parathyroid hormones: Increases, at least during the latter portion of pregnancy.

25-Hydroxyvitamin D: Unchanged.

1,25-Dihydroxyvitamin D: Increases early in gestation and may later increase further.

Calcitonin: Data *conflicting,* with some investigators reporting an increase and others noting no change.

Ovaries and Placenta

Progesterone: Increases markedly from 0.2 μg/ml during the early menstrual cycle to an average of 139 μg/ml by term (i.e., a 1000-fold increase in some women).

Estradiol: Increases about 400-fold from an early menstrual value of 0.05 μg/ml to 18.0 μg/ml by term.

17-Hydroxyprogesterone: Increases to achieve maximum values about week 8, reducing somewhat thereafter but levels remaining well above luteal phase values during the remainder of pregnancy.

Relaxin: *Increases* during pregnancy, indicating continuing function of the corpus luteum.

Estriol: Increases throughout pregnancy, both in serum and 24-hour excretion rates.

Estetrol: Possible index of fetal liver function.

hPL: Increases nearly 5,000-fold by term from 0.002 μU/ml to about 10 μU/ml.

hCG: Increases to reach maximum values between 8 and 10 weeks of pregnancy. Peak values of 93 U/ml are average, with term values averaging 14 U/ml.

PITUITARY GLAND

Some teachers have described the pituitary gland as "the conductor of the hormone orchestra," leaving the impression that, without a pituitary gland, there can be only endocrinologic discord. During pregnancy, however, this is not the case. Maternal hypophysectomy at about 12 weeks of gestation neither disrupts pregnancy nor influences infant outcome adversely, and women who suffer from hypopituitarism and are made to ovulate by drug therapy can have uncomplicated pregnancies.

Anatomy

Knowledge of pituitary mass and cellular consistency inevitably comes from autopsy material and, as such, can hardly be representative of tissue from a normal physiologic population. Nevertheless, such data suggest that the glands of pregnant or recently pregnant women may be 50% heavier than those of average adult males. The enlargement, almost entirely of the anterior lobe, results from a marked increase in the number of prolactin-secreting cells. In nonpregnant adults, such cells account for about 1% of the acidophil population; in pregnant women, as much as 40%.

Prolactin

From a nonpregnancy average of 213 mIU/liter (10.5 ng/ml), prolactin levels increase to term values in excess of 5,000 mIU/liter (250 ng/ml). Unfortunately, the concentrations determined on a large group of women at each week of pregnancy are not normally distributed, and standard deviations cannot be calculated; geometric mean values at each stage of pregnancy are therefore given in Table 4–1 and the range of concentration shown in Figure 4–1.

No definite role for this marked increase in circulating prolactin has yet been discovered. Women who have had a major part of the anterior pituitary gland

Table 4-1. *Mean prolactin concentrations determined longitudinally in women having uncomplicated pregnancies and normal babies*

Serum Prolactin (mIU/liter)	Gestation (weeks)											
	3	*6*	*8*	*10*	*12*	*16*	*20*	*24*	*28*	*32*	*36*	*38*
Mean	224	372	537	631	676	1318	2188	2884	3548	4073	4786	5012
Number	24	26	30	36	36	36	36	36	36	36	36	32

removed for the management of a prolactinoma can maintain a normal pregnancy and labor spontaneously. Although a basal prolactin level appears to be necessary for the initiation of successful breast-feeding, continued lactation is not completely dependent on prolactin. The marked prolactin surges that normally occur in women following suckling by the infant do not occur in mothers without a complete pituitary gland, but they can successfully lactate.

Despite the overall increase in circulating prolactin levels, the usual daily pattern of episodic release with maximal concentrations occurring in the early hours of the morning appears to be maintained. The pituitary also retains its sensitivity to dopaminergic agonists, such as bromocriptine mesylate, that reduce circulating prolactin levels dramatically if prescribed during pregnancy.

It has been suggested that prolactin secretion during pregnancy is stimulated by the increased levels of circulating estrogens. Certainly, estrogen values have increased significantly by the end of the first trimester, suggesting that estradiol is the primary estrogen stimulus. In longitudinal studies during pregnancy, in which both hormones have been regularly determined in the same patients, however,

Fig. 4-1. *Mean and range of prolactin concentrations throughout normal pregnancy.*

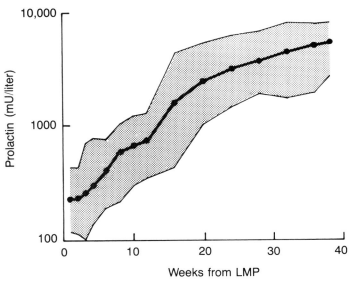

partial correlations do not show any significant relation between the levels of these two hormones.

Prolactin is also present in amniotic fluid at concentrations higher than those in maternal or fetal blood. If pregnant women are given dopamine agonist agents, their circulating prolactin levels and those of the fetus are depressed, but the levels in amniotic fluid are not. It seems probable that the main source for the prolactin in this compartment is the decidua, but the reason for this and the particular role of prolactin around the fetus is uncertain. As fetal skin is freely permeable until approximately 20 weeks' gestation and amniotic fluid is an extension of the fetal extracellular fluid compartment, it is interesting to speculate that prolactin influences fetal salt and water homeostasis, but this remains speculative at the present time.

Follicle-Stimulating Hormone (FSH)

In the normal menstrual cycle, the sex steroids tend to suppress FSH secretion; hence, as could be anticipated, FSH levels are low during pregnancy. Interestingly, postmenopausal women given human chorionic gonadotropin (hCG) also have decreased FSH levels, although their estrogen levels are unaffected; this implies that hCG, too, may have a direct inhibitory effect. Finally, FSH values remain low during lactational amenorrhea when hCG has disappeared from the circulation and estradiol values are much decreased; hence hyperprolactinemia may also play a suppressive role.

Luteinizing Hormone (LH)

Until relatively recently, LH could not be assayed if the concentration of hCG was very high. Now, antibodies specific to the β-subunit of LH have become available, and there seems little doubt that circulating levels of LH are suppressed during normal pregnancy. Absolute values cannot be given, because they depend on the specificity and sensitivity of the assay methods used. In general, however, the low levels found during the luteal phase of the menstrual cycle can be anticipated, and some reports suggest that LH is "undetectable" by term. The fact that "provocation" of the pituitary by LH-releasing hormone has little effect on circulating gonadotropin levels supports the theory that these low levels represent a genuine reduction in secretion rate during pregnancy.

Growth Hormone (hGH)

Concentrations of hGH are reduced during normal pregnancy, but the reason is obscure. Since treatment with estrogens usually increases hGH levels in nonpregnant women, the pregnancy finding is paradoxical. Although some reports suggest a normal hGH response to these stimuli during the first trimester, the usual stimulation of hGH secretion by insulin-induced hypoglycemia or arginine infusion is generally less effective. This blunting or absence of response to these stimuli has been attributed to a suppressive action of human placental lactogen (hPL), but there has been no definitive study to confirm this.

It seems probable that pregnancy can proceed normally without hGH, although data showing this are necessarily rare. One case has been reported in which an ateliotic dwarf (specific deficiency of hGH) had normal pregnancies.

Somatomedin C

The main source of somatomedin C is probably the liver. It has no "gland" of its own, but it has growth-promoting properties and is physiologically tied to the action of growth hormone. Only a few laboratories have been able to purify sufficient of the compound to label it for immunoassay purposes. Thus the available data on somatomedin C levels are limited by the interest of these groups of workers, and the results so far come from a very small data base. They should be interpreted with these marked limitations in mind.

Serum concentrations of somatomedin C appear to be higher in pregnant women at term than in healthy, nonpregnant women, while cord blood concentrations are lower. The timing of this maternal increase in circulating levels has not been pinpointed, but it may occur only during the third trimester. Even the "increase" must be carefully defined in this case; if a mean nonpregnancy concentration is taken to be 1.3 U/ml, the mean value at term is only approximately 1.6 U/ml, with a wide standard deviation. The effect is that some women may have no increase in their somatomedin C values during pregnancy, and a few may even have lower values by term. Many more data are needed before conclusions can be drawn.

Adrenocorticotropic Hormone (ACTH)

A progressive, though modest, increase in maternal serum ACTH is thought to occur throughout pregnancy, with perhaps some decrease by term; again, there is a paradox. Normally, ACTH production by the anterior pituitary is controlled by corticotropin-releasing factor from the hypothalamus. This, in turn, is influenced by circulating cortisol levels; decreased cortisol concentrations stimulate the production of corticotropin-releasing factor and hence ACTH, while high cortisol levels have the opposite effect. During pregnancy, however, ACTH values are increased, despite increased maternal circulating cortisol levels.

It is now known that the placenta produces a substance that is similar to ACTH in its biologic and immunoassayable characteristics. The placenta does not appear to respond to feedback mechanisms, and the ACTH from this nonsuppressible source may account for the increases in circulating maternal cortisol and ACTH.

Thyroid-Stimulating Hormone (TSH)

There are conflicting reports about TSH during pregnancy. Some investigators have suggested that circulating concentrations are increased, while others have found the values to be unchanged. It seems likely that levels are unchanged during pregnancy, because there is a normal rise in TSH concentrations in response to injected thyrotropin-releasing hormone, thyroid suppression by exogenous triiodothyronine (T_3) is normal, and thyroid uptake of radioiodine remains unaltered. (This last test is not recommended because the tracer passes to the fetus.) Pregnancy produces another of its paradoxes here, however; large doses of corticoids suppress plasma TSH concentrations in nonpregnant women, but not in pregnant women.

Melanocyte-Stimulating Hormone (MSH)

A polypeptide, MSH originates from the same prohormone (pro-opiocortin) from which ACTH originates, and levels increase substantially during normal pregnancy—perhaps as much as 100-fold. Fish, reptiles, and amphibians have skin cells called melanophores that contain melanin granules capable of migrating under the influence of α-MSH and β-MSH. Mammals, however, have only melanocyte cells in which the melanin granules do not move. The function of MSH is therefore unclear, and pigmentation associated with endocrine disorders is probably influenced more by ACTH than by MSH. It is possible, however, that the marked increase in MSH during pregnancy is responsible for the characteristic pigmentation of the areolae of the breasts, the adominal linea nigra, and the face (chloasma).

Arginine Vasopressin

Previously called antidiuretic hormone or simply vasopressin, arginine vasopressin originates in specific cells in the hypothalamus and passes to the posterior pituitary gland via the neuronal axons; from there, it is released to the general circulation. By increasing the permeability of the luminal membrane of the collecting tubule cells in the kidney, arginine vasopressin facilitates the reabsorption of water. Osmolality is rigorously maintained in healthy people and a decrease of as little as 2%, or about 6 mosm/kg, suppresses the secretion of arginine vasopressin. Although total osmolality decreases by about 10 mosm/kg during the normal first trimester, the secretion of arginine vasopressin is not permanently suppressed.

Immunoassays for this hormone have been difficult to obtain, and the situation has been made more difficult during pregnancy by the physiologic increase in circulating enzymes (e.g., cystine aminopeptidase) that destroy small polypeptide hormones. Recent data suggest, however, not only that circulating arginine vasopressin concentrations are normal throughout pregnancy, but also that pregnant women respond in the normal way to water deprivation or loading. Thus, it must be concluded that the pregnant woman resets her "osmostat" to a new, lower level (i.e., approximately 280 mosm/kg, rather than the more normal 290 mosm/kg), but that once it has been reset, she guards it by the same physiologic responses made by a nonpregnant woman. Absolute concentrations depend on the laboratory undertaking the assay; in our unit, the normal range is 1 to 3 pg/ml, and this is unaffected by pregnancy.

Oxytocin

Like arginine vasopressin, oxytocin originates in the hypothalamus from specific cells and passes to the posterior pituitary via neuronal axons. The widespread use of synthetic compounds similar to oxytocin to induce labor implies that oxytocin is the "trigger" of spontaneous labor in humans, but such is not the case. Although some reports have suggested that circulating maternal levels of oxytocin increase as spontaneous labor progresses, other researchers have been unable to confirm this. Certainly, there does not appear to be any clear relation between circulating oxytocin concentrations and the strength of the uterine contractions. Levels are markedly increased as the fetal head distends the perineum, but this is specific to that event. Urinary values do not increase during normal labor.

The primary signal for oxytocin release is the stimulation of the nerve endings in the human breast by suckling, which increases intramammary duct pressure and milk ejection; in some instances, temperature change produces a similar response. The same reflex stimulates the release of arginine vasopressin, but this does not appear to be a necessary reaction, because women suffering from diabetes insipidus can breast-feed successfully. Similarly, deliberate water loading of lactating women depresses the level of arginine vasopressin, but not milk ejection. The absence of any increase in intramammary duct pressure during normal labor is further evidence that maternal plasma oxytocin levels do not increase during labor.

THYROID GLAND

During normal pregnancy, the thyroid gland may increase in size, a resting tachycardia develops, the circulation is in a hyperdynamic state, basal metabolic rate increases, and there is often heat intolerance. Thus clinical hyperthyroidism could be diagnosed. In physiological terms, however, the normal pregnant woman has no significant change in her thyroid status.

Anatomy

Although actual histologic evidence must come from autopsy material, with all its inherent limitations, there is little evidence to suggest that there is any change in functional thyroid mass. The increase in size noted in areas where dietary iodine intake is sufficient to prevent endemic goiter is probably due to the increased gland vascularity and the increased amount of stored colloid.

Thyroxine-Binding Globulin (TBG)

The specific circulating protein TBG binds about 85% of all thyroxine (T_4). The major proportion of the remaining 15% is bound to another serum protein, thyroxine-binding prealbumin, and a very small fraction is bound to normal serum albumin. Less than 0.1% exists as free hormone in the circulation, but it is the free fraction that is responsible for all the metabolic activities of the hormone.

The concentrations of TBG have virtually doubled by the end of the first trimester, from a nonpregnancy average of 10 mg/liter to 18 mg/liter (by immunoelectrophoresis). It has been suggested that hepatic stimulation by the increased level of estradiol is responsible for the increase. By the end of the second trimester, the TBG concentration has risen to approximately 24 mg/liter; by term, to 28 mg/liter. In contrast, the value of thyroxine-binding prealbumin is said to decrease somewhat, although again the total circulating amount may be unchanged or even increased when allowance is made for the increase in total blood volume.

T_4, T_3, and rT_3

It is generally accepted that the most important metabolically active factor in the circulation is free T_3; it originates (perhaps as much as 50%) from the peripheral conversion of T_4 and, in this respect, T_4 can be considered a prohormone. The total amount of T_3 is only about one-sixtieth of the amount of T_4. It is less bound to the carrier proteins, however; about 0.5% exists in the free or active state, giving it an effective concentration equal to approximately one-seventh that of free T_4.

The structure of T_4 can be considered a square with an atom of iodine at each corner. During synthesis in the thyroid gland, one atom is incorporated (monoiodotyrosine) and then another (diiodotyrosine). If this cyclic iodination continues, triiodothyronine and thyroxine are formed, the great majority of which is then transported, protein-bound, to peripheral tissues. At the periphery, deiodination can occur, and thyroxine may lose an atom of iodine to become T_3; if it is deiodinated "out of sequence," the resulting compound is still a triiodothyronine, called reverse T_3(rT_3), which is relatively inert (Fig. 4–2). Thus a complex series of events controls the amount of peripherally active T_3.

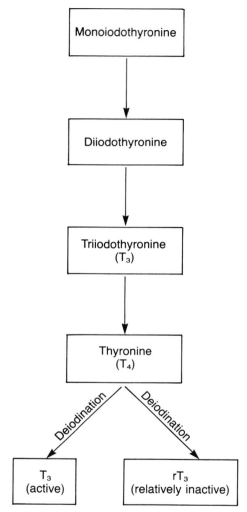

Fig. 4-2. *Formation of T_4, T_3, and rT_3.*

Small amounts of T_4, T_3, and rT_3 can be secreted from the thyroid directly into the circulation, but for all practical purposes, the major proportion of peripherally available hormone arrives bound to protein. Thus, as TBG increases, the concentrations of total T_4 and T_3 also increase if assayed directly; if these were the only laboratory studies conducted on them, all pregnant women would appear to be in a hyperthyroid state. While the available protein-binding sites for T_3 and T_4 are increased, however, they are not saturated; results of other tests, such as the resin uptake of T_3, are low, usually returning the free thyroxine index to the normal range. The majority of sensitive, direct assays of the free hormones suggest that the amounts of free T_4 and T_3 do not change in pregnancy and that the ratio of T_3 to rT_3 is similar to that found in nonpregnant women. However, other investigators have reported the levels of free T_3 and T_4 to be increased, and a recent report from Britain has suggested both values decrease progressively as pregnancy advances!

To try and resolve such conflicts, the amounts of unconjugated T_3 and T_4 in urine have been determined on the theory that such values would reflect the amount of free hormone filtered at the glomerulus. Again, various attempts yield conflicting views, but it seems that the amounts excreted are not increased.

ADRENAL GLANDS

The basic building blocks for the production of steroid hormones are cholesterol and acetate; from these, estrogens and androgens can be manufactured. Only the adrenal cortex has the necessary enzyme systems for the formation of cortisol, however. It is interesting to note that women who have had a bilateral adrenalectomy not only become pregnant, but also usually need little or no increase in the doses of their replacement therapy.

Anatomy

From the limited autopsy data available, it seems that there is no increase in the combined weight of the adrenal glands during pregnancy, and their histologic appearance is unchanged.

Corticosteroid-Binding Globulin (CBG) or Transcortin

The concentration of CBG increases markedly during normal pregnancy, from average values of approximately 20 μg/100 ml to 45 μg/100 ml or more by the second trimester. It appears that hepatic synthesis is increased under the influence of estrogens, since the increase is unaffected by hGH or the thyroid hormones. Approximately 75% of cortisol is bound to CBG, some 15% is bound to albumin, and 10% is free. The bound fractions are metabolically inactive so that, while the proportion of free cortisol is the same during pregnancy, the absolute amount metabolically available is increased. Approximately 10% of aldosterone is also bound to CBG.

Cortisol

By term, circulating concentrations of cortisol are twofold to threefold higher than those of nonpregnant women (i.e., they increase from about 120 μg/liter to about 350 μg/liter). Urinary free cortisol also increases from about 50 to 200 μg or more during the third trimester. It is unlikely that this increase results from a marked increase in adrenal cortisol production; the explanation probably lies in changes in cortisol metabolism and a reduced rate of clearance from the circulation.

The upper end of the normal pregnancy range of both plasma and urinary cortisol concentrations overlaps with the levels found in nonpregnant women with Cushing's disease. Yet pregnant women are not clinically Cushingoid unless their altered response to an oral glucose tolerance test or increased urinary loss of amino acids is attributed to this cause.

The episodic release of cortisol in nonpregnant women (maximum at about 8:00 A.M. and minimum about midnight) has been variously reported to be unchanged in pregnancy or altered so that the midnight values during pregnancy are higher than those in nonpregnant women.

17-ketosteroid excretion may be unaltered by pregnancy or increased slightly because of the metabolites of progesterone. 17-hydroxycorticosteroid excretion is unchanged or may decrease somewhat because of a reduction in the tetrahydro-metabolites of glucocorticoids and the excretion of other products that bypass the formation of 17-hydroxycorticosteroids.

Aldosterone

Circulating levels of aldosterone are at least twofold higher at term than those found in nonpregnant women; sometimes the levels are several times higher. Thus the level for nonpregnant women ranged from 100 to 200 ng/liter, while that for women in late pregnancy ranged from 200 to 700 ng/liter. Unlike the increase in cortisol, the increase in aldosterone appears to be due to a genuine increase in production. Neither the protein binding nor the clearance rate is much altered, but the excretion of aldosterone metabolites increases. Secretion rates for nonpregnant women of about 190 μg/24 hours have been described, compared to 240 to 1,000 μg/24 hours for a group of six women studied late in pregnancy.

The stimulus for the increased aldosterone production is difficult to isolate, if indeed any single factor is responsible. It is known that maternal sodium losses result from the increase in glomerular filtration rate, the effect of progesterone, and fetal demand. Furthermore, renin levels are increased, leading ultimately to increased concentrations of angiotensin II. All these factors are probably responsible for the increased circulating concentrations of aldosterone.

11-Deoxycorticosterone (DOC)

A weak mineralocorticoid hormone, DOC actually shows the biggest proportional increase in circulating levels of all the adrenal steroids; it reaches peak values at term. In nonpregnant women, circulating concentrations have been reported to be 0.1 μg/liter or less, while averaging 2.55 μg/liter in pregnant women close to term. Usually, DOC production is stimulated by ACTH and suppressed by dexamethasone; the fact that this is not so during pregnancy suggests that DOC arises from a site other than the maternal adrenal (e.g., the fetoplacental unit). It is just as likely, however, that it comes from the 21-hydroxylation of maternal progesterone, which is also extraadrenal, and more than 8 mg DOC may be produced each day in this way.

Testosterone

It is difficult to be specific about the significance of any changes in circulating concentrations of testosterone during pregnancy because of its multifocal origin, its apparent metabolism by the placenta, and the increase in circulating levels of the sex hormone–binding globulin. The adrenals can produce small amounts of testosterone directly, but they more commonly produce androstenedione, which is peripherally converted to testosterone. The ovaries, too, secrete testosterone directly. The placenta produces it, but probably metabolizes it locally and directly to estrogens so that little, if any, reaches the maternal circulation. The production rate appears to be unaltered by pregnancy, but the amount available for action is reduced because of the increased binding to sex hormone–binding globulin. Thus total testosterone concentrations are elevated from a nonpregnancy average of 0.49 μg/liter to 1.14 μg/liter, but the free hormone levels decrease from 0.0044 μg/liter to 0.0023 μg/liter during pregnancy.

Androstenedione

Approximately 50% of androstenedione comes from the adrenals and 50% from the ovaries. There appears to be a genuine increase in maternal levels during pregnancy, because concentrations increase from a nonpregnancy average of 1.81 μg/liter to about 2.49 μg/liter during late pregnancy. As it is not bound to sex hormone–binding globulin, it is unaffected by the increase in the level of this binding protein. The most significant effect of pregnancy on the androstenedione level is that its transformation to estradiol and estrone is approximately ten times greater than that in nonpregnant patients.

Dehydroepiandrosterone (DHEA) and the Sulfate (DHEAS)

Some reports suggest that circulating DHEA levels are unaltered during pregnancy, while others report a small decrease, for example, from a nonpregnancy average value of 5.02 μg/liter to 3.63 μg/liter late in pregnancy. Some DHEA may come from the ovaries, but most originates from the adrenals and circulates mainly protein-bound. It is aromatized to estradiol and estrone and may account for up to 9% of circulating estradiol at term.

It seems likely that the blood levels reflect a new point of balance between the formation and the metabolic clearance of DHEA, as both functions work at nearly double their nonpregnancy rates. The situation is somewhat more complex with DHEAS. Maternal levels are only about one-half to one-third the nonpregnancy average, but the metabolic clearance rate is increased about eightfold; thus the new point of balance appears to be an approximately twofold increase in production.

Catecholamines

Such cross-sectional studies of catecholamines as there are suggest that, in an unstressed resting situation, circulating levels of epinephrine, norepinephrine, and dopamine are unaffected by pregnancy; urinary values support this. One recent longitudinal study of epinephrine concentrations throughout pregnancy suggested a small, but definite, decrease within patients, however.

Table 4-2 is a summary of the effects of pregnancy on levels of the aforementioned hormones.

ISLET CELLS OF THE PANCREAS

Because circulating insulin and glucagon concentrations are so markedly affected by meals, it is difficult to describe any specific changes they may undergo

Table 4-2. *Blood levels of the adrenal hormones in some nonpregnant women and others during late pregnancy* *

	Conc. (μg/l)	
Adrenal Hormones	*Nonpregnant*	*Late Pregnancy*
Cortisol	120	350
Aldosterone	1-2	2-7
DOC†	0.1	2.6
Testosterone	0.49	1.14
Androstenedione	1.81	2.49
DHEA	5.02	3.63
Catecholamines	Probably unchanged	
Binding protein		
CBG‡	200	450

*The data refer to total concentrations, but should be taken to indicate the direction and approximate magnitude of change rather than absolute values.
†Deoxycorticosterone
‡Corticosteroid-binding globulin (transcortin)

during pregnancy unless pregnant women are given a standard oral glucose load and blood samples are obtained at specific time intervals thereafter. An alternative is to test each woman after a standardized interval of fasting, but their initial nutritional status must be adequate to ensure that fasting does not evoke starvation rather than fasting responses. Rarely are ideal test circumstances attained, so descriptions of alterations in glucose, insulin, and glucagon responses must be interpreted with this stricture in mind.

Anatomy

It is usually reported that expectant mothers are "hyperinsulinic." Certainly, such human data as are available suggest that the islet cells are hypertrophied, largely because of hyperplasia of the B cells.

Insulin (B Cells)

In the fasted state, insulin levels are unchanged during the first and second trimesters of pregnancy, averaging approximately 5 μU/ml; toward term, there is a small, but statistically significant, increase to an average of about 8 μU/ml. In contrast, fasting blood glucose concentrations decrease significantly during the first trimester, but are unaltered thereafter; this seems to preclude any cause and effect relationship between the changes in fasting glucose and insulin.

Peak insulin levels are achieved approximately 40 minutes after a standard oral glucose load in nonpregnant women; these levels reach an average value of about 42 μU/ml. In pregnant women at term, the maximum concentration is achieved approximately 58 minutes after such a glucose load, attaining values of about 66 μU/ml. After 2 hours, the insulin concentrations of nonpregnant women have returned to the region of their fasting levels, but pregnant women at term still have circulating values of 28 μU/ml or more. Thus, during pregnancy, plasma insulin is maintained at levels well above fasting values for longer periods of time, thus justifying the term *hyperinsulinism* for pregnant women and giving rise to the unfortunate phrase "insulin resistance." This term is too generalized because pregnant women respond to the lipogenic and antilipolytic effects of insulin in the same way as do nonpregnant women. The ultimate result is not hypoglycemia or, indeed, even normoglycemia, because blood glucose levels also remain elevated longer after an oral glucose challenge.

The rate of disappearance of monocomponent insulin injected into fasted pregnant women near term is no different from that found in the same fasted women 12 weeks postdelivery (i.e., a half-life of about 3 to 4 minutes on the average).

Glucagon (A Cells)

Basal glucagon concentrations from 44 pg/ml to 181 pg/ml have been reported. The differing results may be due in part to variations in the specificity and the sensitivity of the assays used to determine glucagon levels, but it seems reasonable to conclude that levels are increased. In one report, glucagon and insulin concentrations were determined in blood samples from the same healthy patients throughout pregnancy. Their fasting glucagon values increased from 118 pg/ml between 16 and 24 weeks to 154 pg/ml by term; their fasting insulin values increased over the same interval. The authors then expressed both values in molar equivalents and divided the insulin value by the glucagon value to obtain the I/G ratio. This increased from a nonpregnancy value of 1.1 ± 0.2 to 1.8 ± 0.4, which is statistically significant and suggests that (in these terms) the basal insulin concentration increases proportionally more than does the basal glucagon concentration. In effect, the liver's response to an increased I/G ratio may be the reason for the increased basal glucagon value.

Somatostatin (D Cells)

Little is known about the secretion of somatostatin during pregnancy. In nonpregnant subjects, its stimulated secretion parallels that of insulin with respect to the effect of glucose, leucine and arginine. Somatostatin inhibits the release of both insulin and glucagon, but whether pancreatic or gastrointestinal somatostatin have any specific role during human pregnancy is unknown.

CALCIUM REGULATION

Calcium metabolism consists of a dynamic relationship between a large pool of calcium in the skeleton and a smaller pool in extracellular fluid. This relationship is regulated by two hormones—parathyroid hormone and calcitonin—and vitamin D, which act on bone to maintain the level of calcium ions in serum within narrow physiologic limits. Parathyroid hormone promotes bone resorption, urinary phosphate excretion, and renal conversion of 25-hydroxyvitamin D (the principal circulating form of the vitamin) to its active metabolite 1,25-dihydroxyvitamin D. Calcitonin exerts generally opposite actions on bone. Thus, parathyroid hormone and vitamin D have hypercalcemic actions whereas calcitonin is hypocalcemic.

The pregnant woman must maintain her serum calcium level in the face of an expanding extracellular fluid volume, increasing calcium excretion by the kidney, and calcium transfer to the fetus. The principal physiologic adjustment made for this purpose is an increased secretion of parathyroid hormone; nearly all studies have found that serum parathyroid hormone levels are elevated during pregnancy, at least during the latter portion. Maternal levels of 25-hydroxyvitamin (D_3) are not affected appreciably by gestation, as they are dependent on dietary intake and amount of exposure to ultraviolet light. Values for the active metabolite 1,25-dihydroxyvitamin D, however, increase throughout gestation and are approximately doubled by term. It is believed that the mechanism involves primarily the increased secretion of parathyroid hormone, but prolactin, hGH, and estrogens may be involved as well.

The effect of pregnancy on calcitonin secretion is less clear. Some investigators have noted an increase in calcitonin levels during pregnancy. Such an increase seems a logical mechanism for protecting the maternal skeleton from excessive resorption in the face of relative hyperparathyroidism, while at the same time permitting the gut and kidney effects of parathyroid hormone to provide extra calcium. Other studies, however, have found no change in maternal calcitonin levels during pregnancy.

OVARIES AND PLACENTA

For many years, it was taught that the corpus luteum of the ovary provided the early endocrinologic support for human pregnancy; after a finite interval (about 56 days), the corpus luteum was thought to regress, and all subsequent sex steroid production was believed to take place in the placenta. It is now known, however, that the corpus luteum continues to produce hormones throughout pregnancy at a rate higher than that of the luteal phase of a normal menstrual cycle.

Progesterone

It is usually stated that progesterone production originates in the corpus luteum over the first 7 to 8 weeks of pregnancy; that the placenta then takes over production; and that, even if the corpus luteum is surgically removed, pregnancy continues. This latter observation is certainly true. The removal of the corpus luteum does not interrupt a pregnancy after about 8 weeks of gestation, but the corpus luteum does continue to function if left in place.

The serum progesterone values obtained from a group of women followed throughout pregnancy, beginning in the conceptual month, show that the average luteal concentration achieved at week 4 does not increase until approximately week 12 (Table 4–3, Fig. 4–3). This plateau effect is evident in individuals and is not a statistical quirk. Interpretation is difficult, but the data appear to indicate two possibilities: 1) the placenta does not contribute a great deal to progesterone levels before week 10; or 2) if the placenta is increasing production of this hormone, the increase is balanced by a decreased output by the corpus luteum. The same is not true of estradiol production, and further data are needed to clarify this unusual situation.

Table 4-3. *Longitudinal study of various ovarian and placental hormones throughout pregnancy* *

Gestation (weeks)	Progesterone (µg/ml)		Estradiol (µg/ml)		hPL (µU/ml)		hCG (U/ml)		17-OH Prog (ng/ml)	
	Mean	Range	Mean	Range	Mean	Range	Mean	Range	Mean	Range
1	0.2	0.2–0.6	0.05	0.03–0.16	—	—	—	—	—	—
2	0.6	0.2–22.5	0.07	0.03–0.18	—	—	—	—	—	—
3	8.2	5.2–33.3	0.11	0.05–0.32	0.002	0–0.01	—	—	—	—
4	20.4	11.9–35.5	0.13	0.03–0.41	0.002	0–0.01	0.042	0–11.5	5.8	3.5–10.4
6	20.4	5.3–45.5	0.31	0.12–0.88	0.004	0–0.02	13.2	1.6–67.1	7.0	4.2–12.5
8	21.4	11.3–39.7	0.65	0.24–2.8	0.041	0.002–0.18	71.8	10–242	5.7	3.6–9.6
10	24.2	9.1–56.4	1.03	0.20–2.9	0.22	0.019–0.61	93.3	38–216	3.3	3.3–9.7
12	26.7	12.8–58.2	1.4	0.32–3.9	0.58	0.17–1.5	61.0	21–144	3.9	2.7–7.9
16	34.4	15.6–64.0	3.1	0.93–7.3	1.7	0.85–2.9	23.2	7.8–90		
20	44.1	21.5–85.7	5.6	2.3–14.7	2.5	1.4–4.5	13.2	5.4–35		
24	63.0	31.9–114.3	8.3	3.7–17.9	4.0	2.1–8.4	9.6	2.6–32		
28	81.8	39.1–200.0	10.2	3.4–24.3	5.7	3.2–9.3	9.8	2.8–37		
32	101.9	42.8–230.7	11.2	4.6–26.1	7.8	4.0–15.4	11.6	2.4–50		
36	122.5	40.3–277.3	14.8	5.0–33.5	9.6	4.9–19.1	14.8	2.8–69		
38	138.7	48.3–397.2	18.0	7.3–37.2	9.6	4.8–21.0	13.7	2.5–79		

* As the distribution of these hormones at each stage of pregnancy was skewed, geometric means and ranges are given rather than standard deviations. **Key:** hPL, human placental lactogen; hCG, human chorionic gonadotrophin; 17-OH prog, 17 hydroxyprogesterone.

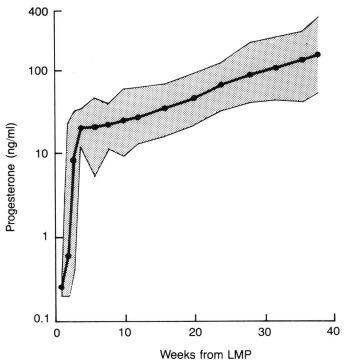

Fig. 4-3. *Serum progesterone values (mean and range) throughout normal pregnancy; note the log scale for concentration.*

Estradiol

The circulating concentration of estradiol increases progressively as gestation advances, and there is no evidence of any plateau effect similar to that of progesterone (Table 4–2, Fig. 4–4). Thus there is a constantly changing relationship between the concentrations of progesterone and estradiol. In the follicular phase of a menstrual cycle, the ratio of progesterone to estradiol is approximately 5:1, expressing both in picograms per milliliter. During the luteal phase, the marked increase in progesterone causes the ratio to increase to as much as 150:1 or more, and this is the relationship at conception. By 12 weeks, the ratio has decreased to approximately 20:1 because of the relative stability of progesterone values while the value of estradiol continues to increase. Both hormone levels increase thereafter, but the relatively greater increase in estradiol causes the ratio to decrease to approximately 8:1 by 36 weeks. It is interesting to note that, if luteectomy is performed prior to approximately 8 weeks, pregnancy can be maintained by the administration of exogenous progesterone alone, but not estradiol alone.

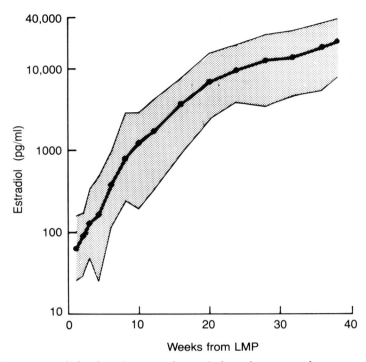

Fig. 4-4. *Serum estradiol values (mean and range) throughout normal pregnancy; note the log scale for concentration.*

17-Hydroxyprogesterone

For all practical purposes, the serum levels of 17-hydroxyprogesterone can be attributed to the corpus luteum, and the increase during early pregnancy reflects increasing corpus luteum function. Peak values occur about week 8 of gestation; the concentrations decrease somewhat thereafter, but remain at levels in excess of menstrual cycle levels through the end of pregnancy (Table 4–2). Some investigators have described a secondary increase in circulating concentrations toward term.

Relaxin

The structure of relaxin has a marked similarity to that of both insulin and the somatomedins, so relaxin may have "growth-promoting" qualities. Its name, however, is derived from its ability to relax ligaments, the cervix, and perhaps even myometrial contractility. In women it appears to arise exclusively from the ovaries, specifically the corpus luteum; thus, like the level of 17-OH progesterone, the level of relaxin should indicate the level of activity of the corpus luteum throughout pregnancy.

Because assays vary in sensitivity and specificity, absolute concentrations are open to question. It seems probable, however, that levels are elevated throughout pregnancy, because they decrease sharply if luteectomy is performed at the time of cesarean delivery. If term values are 0.6 ng/ml to 1.6 ng/ml, concentrations are 0.2 ng/ml or less by 48 hours postoperation.

The timing of the pregnancy increase is difficult to determine. Some reports suggest that it is maximal by the end of the first trimester and maintained thereafter; others, that it increases progressively as gestation advances. In some assays, relaxin cannot be detected during the luteal phase of normal menstrual cycles, raising a question as to whether this is due to lack of assay sensitivity or whether the hormone is specific to pregnancy.

Estriol

Estradiol and estrone are synthesized by the placenta from DHEA that is obtained from both the mother and the fetus. Estriol is synthesized by the placenta largely from 16α-hydroxydehydroepiandrosterone sulfate originating in the fetus. The fetal precursor is its adrenal DHEAS, which can reach the metabolic pathway via the fetal liver (the dominant route) or via the placenta. Maternal adrenal DHEAS can also contribute via the placental–fetal liver pathway so that, while the estriol level reflects fetal metabolism primarily, it is not doing so exclusively.

Until the advent of immunoassay methods, the blood levels of estriol were too low to be measured accurately, and most researchers reported 24-hour urinary amounts. These increase from approximately 2 mg/24 hours by the end of the first trimester to approximately 30 mg/24 hours by term. Plasma levels increase from about 56 μg/liter at midpregnancy to an average of 250 μg/liter at term. Unfortunately, there is considerable variation not only in different patients, but also in the same patient from day to day and even from time of day to time of day. The elegance and precision of immunoassay techniques have revealed the pitfalls of using such levels to interpret fetal well-being. Urinary output covered a longer period and inevitably blunted much of this physiologic variation. The very bluntness of the tool detracted from its clinical usefulness, however.

Estetrol

Largely derived from the 15α- and 16α-hydroxylation of estriol by the fetal liver, estetrol may be an index of fetal liver function. Few data are available, however.

Human Placental Lactogen (hPL)

Of the 191 amino acids that make up hPL, 162 are identical to those of human growth hormone (hGH). Furthermore, hPL is chemically similar to human prolactin. It might be anticipated therefore that hPL has growth-promoting properties, but it has proved difficult to discover any actual function for this placental protein hormone. The fact that detectable amounts of the hormone appear in the maternal circulation some 7 to 10 days postconception indicates an incredible amount of metabolic work by the early embryonic tissue, and the continuing rapid increase thereafter seems to imply a very basic and fundamental role (Table 4–2). Even with this physiologic argument, however, its actual role remains speculative.

Obviously, hPL cannot be withdrawn during pregnancy, so tests must be conducted by giving the hormone to nonpregnant subjects. This is a poor model, because the rest of the hormonal milieu of these subjects is inappropriate for pregnancy; the conclusions drawn from such studies are unsatisfactory at best. It could be argued that, as this hormone is of fetal origin but goes almost exclusively into the maternal circulation, it has some role as a signal to the mother. Conversely, it may have an entirely local action around the site of placental implantation, and its passage into the maternal circulation may be merely the method by which it is removed from that site.

Recently, it has been shown that log values of the concentrations of hPL over the first 14 weeks of pregnancy have a linear relation to the number of days of gestation.

Human Chorionic Gonadotropin (hCG)

A glycoprotein placental hormone, hCG is composed of two subunits, α and β. The α subunit is nearly identical to the α subunit of LH, TSH, and FSH, while the β subunit has some similarities to that of LH. It was this close similarity that made the assay of LH during pregnancy so difficult in the presence of overwhelming amounts of hCG.

Again, the metabolic power displayed by the developing embryo in producing hormone in assayable amounts within 6 days or so of conception is impressive. The hCG concentration increases rapidly thereafter, reaching peak values between weeks 8 and 10 and declining somewhat thereafter (Table 4–2, Fig. 4–5). A small secondary rise occurs in some, but not all, women between 32 and 38 weeks of gestation; this may be related to fetal sex, as many women who showed this secondary increase had female infants.

The role of hCG is more clearly defined than that of hPL. The human corpus luteum contains specific high affinity receptors for hCG, and injections of this hormone maintain the life of the corpus luteum in nonpregnant women. It may also enhance the production of progesterone in the corpus luteum and the conversion of cholesterol to pregnanolone in the placenta. The fetal adrenal synthesis of DHEA

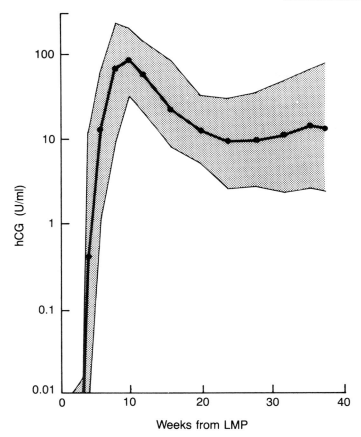

Fig. 4-5. *Serum hCG values (mean and range) throughout normal pregnancy; note the log scale for concentration.*

and fetal testicular secretion of testosterone may be influenced by the level of hCG. An immunosuppressive function that helps the pregnant woman to "tolerate" her fetus has been described, but has not gained universal support; others have suggested that this function may actually be due to other factors present in "impure" hCG preparations.

As with hPL, there is a log linear relationship between hCG blood concentrations and day of gestation until approximately 56 days. If the early placental cells work at a set production rate per cell, this relationship would provide an index of increasing placental cell numbers over this early phase of fetal development. Indeed, a highly accurate method of determining the length of human pregnancy from the concentrations of hPL and hCG has been described and may become one of the most useful clinical functions of these hormones.

5

Respiratory System

Anatomy and Functional Components

Subcostal angle: Increases from about 68° to 103° causing an increase of approximately 2 cm in the transthoracic diameter.

Tidal volume: Increases by about 200 ml or 40%.

Expiratory reserve volume: Decreases by approximately 200 ml.

Residual volume: Decreases by some 300 ml or 20%.

Vital capacity: May be increased, but few serial data are available.

Inspiratory capacity: Appears to *increase* by about 300 ml.

Functional residual volume: Decreases by as much as 500 ml.

Minute volume: Increases by about 40% or 3 liters/min.

Maximum Breathing Capacity: Is *unaffected.*

Forced expiratory volume: Appears to be *unaffected.*

Peak expiratory flow rate: Also appears to be *unaffected.*

Closing volume: May increase.

Pulmonary diffusing capacity: Probably *decreases* by approximately 4 ml/min/mm Hg (carbon monoxide).

Oxygen requirement
Increases by 30 to 40 ml/min.

Carbon dioxide output
Expressed as the respiratory quotient, probably *increases.*

Carbon dioxide pressure
Markedly *decreases* in range from 35 to 40 mm Hg to 28 to 30 mm Hg.

Oxygen pressure
Increases by a smaller proportion (i.e., from 85 mm Hg to approximately 92 mm Hg).

pH
Arterial value *unchanged* at 7.4.

Compensatory Physiologic Changes

ANATOMY AND FUNCTIONAL COMPONENTS

Physiologic data are available concerning the respiratory system during pregnancy because noninvasive techniques make it possible to study living normal pregnant women. The angle between the bottom ribs, the **subcostal angle**, increases from the usual 68° or so to approximately 103° by term. The increase, which appears to be progressive, begins long before the uterus is large enough to cause any direct pressure effect, so this rib splaying is a true physiologic response. In some women, the angle never quite returns to its prepregnancy size.

Despite many anecdotal suggestions that the diaphragm is "splinted" by increasing uterine size, this is not true; the diaphragmatic excursion increases by 1 to 2 cm from a nonpregnancy average of approximately 4.5 cm to a term value of 5.5 to 6 cm. The resting level is higher by as much as 4 cm, but the transverse diameter of the thoracic cage increases by up to 2 cm, compensating for this. Far from being less effective, the diaphragm dominates respiration, and the relaxed abdominal musculature plays less of a role.

The lungs appear to be more dense on radiographic pictures, with the lung markings more prominent. This is partly because they collapse more fully during expiration and partly because blood flow is increased in the pulmonary vessels.

The components of pulmonary function are defined in the following manner.

Tidal volume: the volume of air breathed in (or out) during normal respiration with the patient quietly at rest.

Expiratory and inspiratory reserve volume: the maximum volumes breathed out (or in) after normal, rested respiration. Anyone, after having breathed out normally, can force a further volume of gas from the lungs. Similarly, if required, additional air can be breathed in after normal inspiration.

Residual volume: the volume of air remaining in the lung spaces after expiration.

Vital capacity: the maximum total volume of air that can be breathed out after a maximal, forced inspiration. It is thus tidal lung capacity less the residual volume.

89

Inspiratory capacity: the maximum volume of air that can be inspired following a normal, rested expiration; it can be expressed as the tidal volume plus the inspiratory reserve volume.

Functional residual capacity: the amount of air left in the lungs at the end of a normal, rested expiration; it can be expressed as the expiratory reserve volume plus the residual volume. Thus, during resting respiration, this is the "basal" volume of air with which newly inspired air must mix and diffuse to reach the circulation.

Minute volume: the volume of air breathed in (or out) per minute; it can be expressed as tidal volume times the respiratory rate, as this rate is expressed per minute.

The following expressions describe normal physiologic occurrences and must be expanded to embrace specific tests of respiratory function:

Maximum breathing capacity (MBC): the maximum volume of air that can be achieved by forced breathing over 15 seconds. A genuine forced maximal effort is exhausting, and volunteers for this test are therefore scarce, especially during pregnancy.

Forced expiratory volume (FEV): the amount of air that can be forcibly expired in 1 second. It can be expressed either as volume or as a proportion of the vital capacity.

Peak expiratory flow rate (PFR): the peak flow rate achievable during forced expiration. It can be measured directly with a flow meter.

Closing volume (CV): the volume at which the air from the apices, where air entering the lungs goes first but leaves last, begins to appear. It is measured from inhalation of a bolus of foreign gas.

Pulmonary diffusing capacity (PDC): the rate at which different gases diffuse from the alveoli to the blood, expressed as milliliters per minute per millimeter of mercury pressure.

During pregnancy, tidal volume increases from the average nonpregnancy value of 500 ml/min to approximately 700 ml/min, equivalent to an increase of about 40%. Respiratory rate is usually unchanged from about 15 breaths/min so that the minute volume also increases by about 40%, from a little over 7 liters/min to approximately 10 liters/min.

By term, the expiratory reserve volume has been reduced from about 1,300 ml to 1,100 ml, the lower value probably being achieved slowly and progressively. The increased depth of respiration obvious in many expectant mothers is at the expense of this reserve; indeed, the improved ventilation achieved by pregnant women is due to the increased depth of respiration and not its rate.

As pregnancy advances, residual volume decreases progressively from approximately 1,500 ml to 1,200 ml by late pregnancy (i.e., about 20%). Because the tidal volume increases so much and the residual volume with which it must mix is reduced, there is a marked increase in efficiency of gas mixing in the lungs.

Early reports suggested that there was no change in vital capacity during pregnancy from the nonpregnancy average of about 3 liters. Control studies were often undertaken on women only 3 months or less postpartum, however, and these women may not be representative of nonpregnant women. Furthermore, the numbers of patients studied were small. Within the described groups, some women showed marked increases, while others displayed little or no change. Recent serial studies have shown a marked increase in vital capacity during pregnancy, but others have failed to confirm this. It may be that there are wide variations across subjects; more data are needed.

The development of more advanced techniques has caused investigators to reappraise older studies, which suggested that inspiratory capacity did not change in pregnancy or that any increase was of a modest order. It seems probable that inspiratory capacity increases progressively throughout pregnancy, reaching a maximum of approximately 300 ml above nonpregnancy volumes by term.

As both the residual volume and the expiratory reserve volume are reduced, the functional residual capacity made up of these two parts is considerably reduced: probably by as much as 500 ml.

The maximum breathing capacity (MBC) test is no longer used, but such data as are available suggest that it is unaffected by pregnancy.

Forced expiratory volume (FEV) also appears to be unaffected by pregnancy. Most healthy individuals can expire about 85% of their vital capacity in 1 second if asked to do so, and so can pregnant women.

The peak expiratory flow rate appears to be unaffected by pregnancy.

Few data on the closing volumes of normal healthy women are available, and more are needed. One report suggested that the closing volume is increased during pregnancy, but nearly half the women studied had hypertensive complications in their pregnancy and may not be representative.

The higher partial pressure of oxygen in alveolar air, together with the increased efficiency of mixing, might be expected to improve the rate of diffusion across the alveolar membrane. Measurements of gas diffusion show the reverse, however. One study showed a reduction in carbon monoxide diffusion from 26.5 ml/min/mm Hg in nonpregnant women to 22.5 ml/min/mm Hg in women in late pregnancy. This may be due to the lower hemoglobin concentration common in pregnant women during the last trimester or to changes in the capillary vessels surrounding the alveoli that slow the rate of diffusion.

OXYGEN REQUIREMENT

Maternal adaptations to pregnancy in cardiac, renal, and respiratory performance account for approximately two-thirds of the extra oxygen need in pregnancy. The fetus also makes an oxygen demand, but its needs are relatively modest because it does not need to regulate its own temperature. It can be calculated that the extra metabolic activity of pregnancy requires oxygen in the amount of 30 to 40 ml/min or about 15% above nonpregnancy needs. Direct measurements of oxygen consumption not only are difficult and time-consuming, but also require considerable patient cooperation if they are to be undertaken serially. Studies that have been done yield somewhat conflicting data. One report suggested an increase from 191 ml/min to 249 ml/min, while another described an increase from 254 ml/min to 296 ml/min. Despite such differences, there is total accord that an increase does indeed occur and that it is on the order of 30 to 40 ml/min.

CARBON DIOXIDE OUTPUT

The determination of carbon dioxide output is complex, since carbon dioxide does not have to be exhaled immediately, but may be "stored" as bicarbonate in the blood. Attempts have been made to study the relation of carbon dioxide exhaled to oxygen inhaled—the respiratory quotient (RQ). To be reasonably accurate, however, this would have to be determined on patients continuously over several hours and would be affected by the type of food eaten previously (i.e., carbohydrate or lipid). Such limited data as are available suggest that the RQ increases during normal pregnancy.

CARBON DIOXIDE PRESSURE

There is a dramatic decrease in P_{CO_2} from a nonpregnancy range of 35 to 40 mm Hg to 28 to 30 mm Hg during pregnancy. That this is a deliberate adaptation can be easily demonstrated. A nonpregnant woman hyperventilates if made to rebreathe her expired air, and increases of approximately 1.5 liters/min occur for each increase of 1 mm Hg in P_{CO_2}. A pregnant woman shows an increase of 6 liters/min for the same duress. Interestingly, women living at a high altitude already have a lower P_{CO_2} than do those living at sea level, but the P_{CO_2} decreases further when these women become pregnant. This pregnancy reduction is almost certainly an effect of progesterone; it even occurs in a minor way during the luteal phase of each menstrual cycle.

OXYGEN PRESSURE

As would be anticipated from the decrease in P_{CO_2}, there is an increase in P_{O_2} during pregnancy. Data demonstrating this are limited, however. One study reported a rise from 85 mm Hg during the first trimester to 92 mm Hg by term.

pH

For all practical purposes, maternal arterial pH is unaltered from the normal average of 7.4. The implication is that the decrease in PCO_2, which should lead to alkalosis, is matched by a decrease in blood bicarbonate.

COMPENSATORY PHYSIOLOGIC CHANGES

Not all the physiologic changes that occur in pregnant women occur to achieve a specific purpose; some are compensatory, offsetting unwanted side effects from the major changes. The respiratory system offers an excellent example of a possible sequence of checks and balances.

The developing fetus must offload its carbon dioxide into the mother, and this could be achieved in two ways. The fetus could exist in utero at a PCO_2 higher than the mother's or the mother could reduce her basal PCO_2 status. As described earlier, the latter is nature's choice. To achieve this, the mother "overbreathes" to wash out her PCO_2. Because this would normally lead to alkalosis, she compensates by excreting more bicarbonate via the renal system, excreting with it some obligatory sodium. Unfortunately, sodium is a major determinant of plasma osmolality, so this decreases. Lowering osmolality normally causes a diuresis, so the mother's hypothalamic osmoreceptor centers must be reset to accept and guard this lower value. Thus, the primary need to lower maternal PCO_2 initiates a series of events that affect the respiratory and renal systems, as well as significantly altering plasma biochemistry.

Of course, the argument could be purely teleologic, an explanation deliberately embracing the known changes into a plausible whole. It may be possible to think of physiologic arguments showing that this hypothesis is flawed.

6

Alimentary System

Appetite

Usually *increases,* although it can take bizarre forms.

Gastric reflux

Probably caused by a *combination of cardiac sphincter laxity* and some *anatomic displacement.*

Gastric secretion

Decreases in terms of acidity, but mucous production may be increased.

Gastric motility

Almost certainly *decreases.*

Intestinal absorption

Efficiency of absorption may be *increased,* either by specific mechanisms or by a delay in transit time that allows more time for digestion and absorption.

Intestinal transit time

Appears to be *slower* during pregnancy.

Large intestine

Absorption efficiency appears to be *greater* during pregnancy and transit time probably *slower.*

Liver

In functional terms, probably *unchanged,* with normal levels of serum bilirubin.

Gallbladder

May be *passively dilated* and hence larger, but the composition of the bile itself appears to be *unchanged.*

The most fundamental adaptation that women must make during pregnancy is to absorb the extra nutrients and minerals needed for the development of a healthy fetus. Yet, although the gastrointestinal tract is relatively accessible, compared, for example, to the heart or kidneys, few physiologic data are available.

APPETITE

That energy demand is increased during pregnancy cannot be doubted. The pregnant woman can meet this need by conserving energy used in nonessential ways or by increasing her food intake. Individual women use both methods, achieving their own balance. In general, pregnant women do rest more, make less extravagant limb gestures, and otherwise conserve energy by avoiding nonessential movement; their physicians may encourage them in this attitude. Pregnant women seem to have a significant increase in appetite as well. This usually leads to a generally increased intake of all types of food, while their physicians emphasizes those foods of greatest nutritional, vitamin, and mineral value.

In some cases, the urge to eat takes bizarre forms. Pregnant women may experience a craving for things such as coal, toothpaste, soap, strongly spiced or pickled foods, and even disinfectant liquids. They may develop powerful aversions to otherwise normal foods, such as coffee, tea, or chocolate. The obstetrician is unlikely to be aware of these changes, because patients rarely volunteer such information and often deny such cravings, even if asked directly; indeed, even their husbands are usually unaware of their cravings. Such habits in themselves are unlikely to cause any adverse effect, but such things as coal and clay have a powerful adsorption and buffering capacity and could, if taken in excess, reduce the absorption of minerals and vitamins from the gut.

In contrast, some women experience a reduction in appetite. During early pregnancy, this may be associated with a feeling of nausea; during late pregnancy, it may be caused by reflux esophagitis (heartburn). Attention to these symptoms usually improves appetite. Some women, however, genuinely lose their desire to eat, which can, although rarely, lead to the extreme of anorexia nervosa.

GASTRIC REFLUX

Epigastric burning pain caused by the passage of gastric acid into the lower esophagus is so common that it is regarded as normal by many pregnant women. Among the suggested causes of this are a reduction of lower esophageal (cardiac) sphincter tone, increased intraabdominal pressure, mechanical displacement of the lower esophageal sphincter, and even hiatus herniation (displacement of the sphincter into the thoracic cavity). It has even been suggested that the symptoms cannot be attributed exclusively to gastric acidity. Some women studied by means of a pH electrode in the esophagus had a change in pH, but no symptoms, while others with symptoms had no change in pH. Whatever the explanation, management with an antacid preparation is usually effective, improving appetite and hence nutrient intake.

GASTRIC SECRETION

Acid production appears to be considerably reduced during early and midpregnancy after a period of fasting, after the ingestion of water or saline, or after the administration of histamine; it regains or exceeds nonpregnancy rates by term. Thus a secretion rate in nonpregnant women of 63 ± 7.8 mg/45 min reportedly decreased to 36 ± 12 mg/45 min by the second trimester, but reached 107 ± 20 mg/45 min late in pregnancy. There is usually considerable variation between individuals, however, and the amount of neutralizing mucous secretion in the stomach is also a factor. Blood pepsin levels, which reflect gastric secretion, show a similar pattern of change during pregnancy.

GASTRIC MOTILITY

The nature of the methods that may be used to investigate gastric motility in pregnancy makes data difficult to obtain and to interpret. Using radiopaque dyes so that gastric emptying can be visualized is not practical on a serial basis, and the nature of such liquids may itself affect the speed of emptying. The need to recover other forms of dyed liquids at set intervals following their oral ingestion necessitates intubation, which is not only unpleasant, but also may affect the normal physiology. Finally, the composition of the ingested material may influence its speed of transit through the stomach. If the stomach is indeed an "atonic bag" with a lax duodenal sphincter, water or isotonic saline may literally flow through it without any muscular motility on the part of the stomach walls; if hypertonic solutions, such as glucose, are taken, the osmolality may inhibit emptying. Finally, most nutrients are semisolid and may have different emptying characteristics from those of fluids.

These difficulties make it imprudent to give absolute figures, but the evidence suggests a reduction in gastric motility and a delay in complete emptying time during pregnancy. This is probably further reduced during labor; physicians who administer general anesthetics to women in labor have found it clinically prudent to expect the complete emptying time to be almost double the emptying time in nonpregnant women (i.e., 75 minutes in nonpregnant patients and 120 minutes in women during late pregnancy).

INTESTINAL ABSORPTION

Nutrients are absorbed at a given rate across the walls of the appropriate sections of the intestines. The apparently increased absorption efficiency during pregnancy could be a physiologic adjustment involving specific mechanisms to improve the rate, or it could be the result of a slower transit time through the gut that allows more time for absorption at the normal rate. Again, data are necessarily limited, but it seems that the absorption of iron and calcium is probably improved by specific mechanisms. The understandably limited data obtained from women who have undergone pregnancies following the surgical removal of large sections of their small bowel or bypass operations, such as jejunoileostomy, suggest that their stools are less frequent and better formed with a smaller fat content during pregnancy, however.

INTESTINAL TRANSIT TIME

Transit times have been measured in healthy women who swallowed a tube loaded with a small mercury-containing balloon. The mean time from swallowing to cecum was 57.9 ± 12.1 hours in pregnant women and 51.7 ± 9.6 hours in nonpregnant women. It seems highly unlikely that such intervals reflect the passage of food; presumably, they indicate the unphysiologic nature of forcing a tube down the intestinal lumen. They do, however, indicate a reduced gut motility during pregnancy.

A much more physiologic study can be conducted by giving women levulose to drink; when it reaches the cecum, bacterial action rapidly releases hydrogen that can be detected in the expired breath by highly sensitive electrodes. Such studies suggest that the normal transit time for such liquids increases from the usual 90 minutes to between 150 and 200 minutes in pregnant women during the last trimester.

LARGE INTESTINE

Few data are available concerning absorption efficiency and motility of the large bowel. In one study, a tube with a mercury balloon at its tip was swallowed by pregnant women. When it eventually reached the ileocecal valve, solutions were introduced at the rate of 24 ml/min and the absorption rates for water and sodium determined. In nonpregnant women, the rate for water was 1.16 ml/min, and the rate for sodium was 323 μEq/min. During the first half of pregnancy, these rates increased to 1.84 ml/min and 470 μEq/min, respectively.

Motility data, which are largely anecdotal, are concerned with the incidence of constipation during pregnancy. While it seems to be generally accepted that constipation is more common during pregnancy, presumably reflecting a reduced transit time and increased removal of water, agreement is not universal. A report from Israel in which 1,000 healthy women were questioned postdelivery about their bowel habit showed that about 55% reported no change, 34% an increased stool frequency, and only 11% a decrease.

LIVER

Blood bilirubin concentrations remain in the normal nonpregnancy range in uncomplicated pregnancies, and it is generally agreed that liver function is unaffected in terms of the usual biochemical tests. The clearance of the injected dye Bromsulphalein (BSP) from the circulation has been investigated most thoroughly. The usual sequence of events is for the dye to be removed from the blood by the liver, conjugated, and passed into the bile. During normal pregnancy, the rate of removal is slowed, but this could be the result of other mechanisms. For example, a delayed excretion from the liver to bile may cause the dye to pass from the liver to the blood, competition by the increased level of estrogens for liver binding sites may displace BSP, and increased avidity by the binding plasma proteins may reduce uptake by the liver.

GALLBLADDER

Radiographic studies suggest that the motility of the gallbladder is reduced during pregnancy. When egg yolk and milk were used to provoke emptying of the gallbladder in pregnant women, it was found that some women had discharged only 38% of the gallbladder's contents 40 minutes later, while the same women 6 to 8 weeks postdelivery discharged 71% over the same time interval. Direct examination of the gallbladder at cesarean delivery also indicates a degree of dilatation and atony in about 75% of women at this time. While there is anecdotal evidence that gallstones are more frequent during pregnancy, the data available on the actual composition of the bile suggests that it is unchanged during pregnancy.

Index